THE STORY OF MEDICINE AND DISEASE
IN
MALAŴI

THE 150 YEARS SINCE LIVINGSTONE

MICHAEL and ELSPETH KING

The Story of Medicine and Disease in Malawi

ISBN Number 978-99908-900-0-6

Artwork by Michael King

The authors regret any errors that may have been
included. The opinions expressed are their own.

First Impression May 1992
Second Impression October 1992
Third Impression July 1997

Fourth Impression (facsimile) with added chapters
February 2007

Typeset in Palatino by the MCC, PO Box 205, Blantyre, Malawi
Printed in Blantyre by The Montfort Press
and by Victoire Press in Cambridge, England

Copies available at Daunt Books, London:
orders@dauntbooks.com
and at Heffers Bookshop, Cambridge
medical@heffers.co.uk

and at
www.Amazon.co.uk

Acknowledgements

We would like to thank: The Ministry of Health; the Government Censorship Board; the Polytechnic Blantyre, the University of Malawi, the Livingstonia Synod, Malawi, the National National Archives, Zomba, the National Library Service of Malawi, the Museums of Malawi at Blantyre, Mangochi and Mzuzu; the Society of Malawi Library, Blantyre; Mlambe and Likuni Mission Hospitals; Nkhoma Mission Hospital; the White Fathers, Malawi.

We are very grateful to: the Rev. Peter and Vera Garland, Tom and Jennifer Gilling, Frank Johnston, Dr. C. Blignaut, Sister Anne Neilson.

We acknowledge assistance of: the British Museaum Library, London; Cambridge University Library; the Wellcome Trust Library, London; Rhodes House, Oxford; the British Council.

We thank the Beit Trust for a grant and our local sponsors: Pharmanova Blantyre, Stagecoach Malawi Ltd; Lonrho Malawi Ltd; Old Mutual, Blantyre; National Bank of Malawi; Sugar Corporation of Malawi Ltd; Oil Company of Malawi Ltd; Ethanol Company Ltd; Hogg Robinson (Malawi) Ltd.

Their generosity will enable this book to reach a wider readership within Malawi, either by subsidy or by presentation through various agencies to Hospital, School and other libraries.

The fourth reprinting (facsimile) has allowed us to add two more chapters, bringing the story up to date. It is now 150 years since David Livingstone started to organize the Zambesi Expedition, which led to him visiting Lake Malawi in 1859.

**To the Clinical Officers and Medical Assistants of Malawi
who for so long have been the backbone of the
Medical Services**

Michael S. King O.B.E., M.A. (Cantab), F.R.C.S. (England), Fellow of
the College of Surgeons of East, Central and   Southern Africa,
Malawi Silver Jubilee Medal 1989.
Chief Surgeon, Queen Elizabeth Hospital, Blantyre 1976-94
Volunteer Surgeon in North Malawi 1995-2007

Elspeth King B.A. Ph.D (London) his wife.
University Lecturer at the Polytechnic Blantyre 1980-94

They have published in the year 2000
"The Great Rift - Africa, Surgery AIDS, Aid"
ISBN 978-09539290-0-9

and in 2007

"AIDS, Surgery and Life - a Malawi Mosaic"
ISBN 978-09539290-1-6

Contents

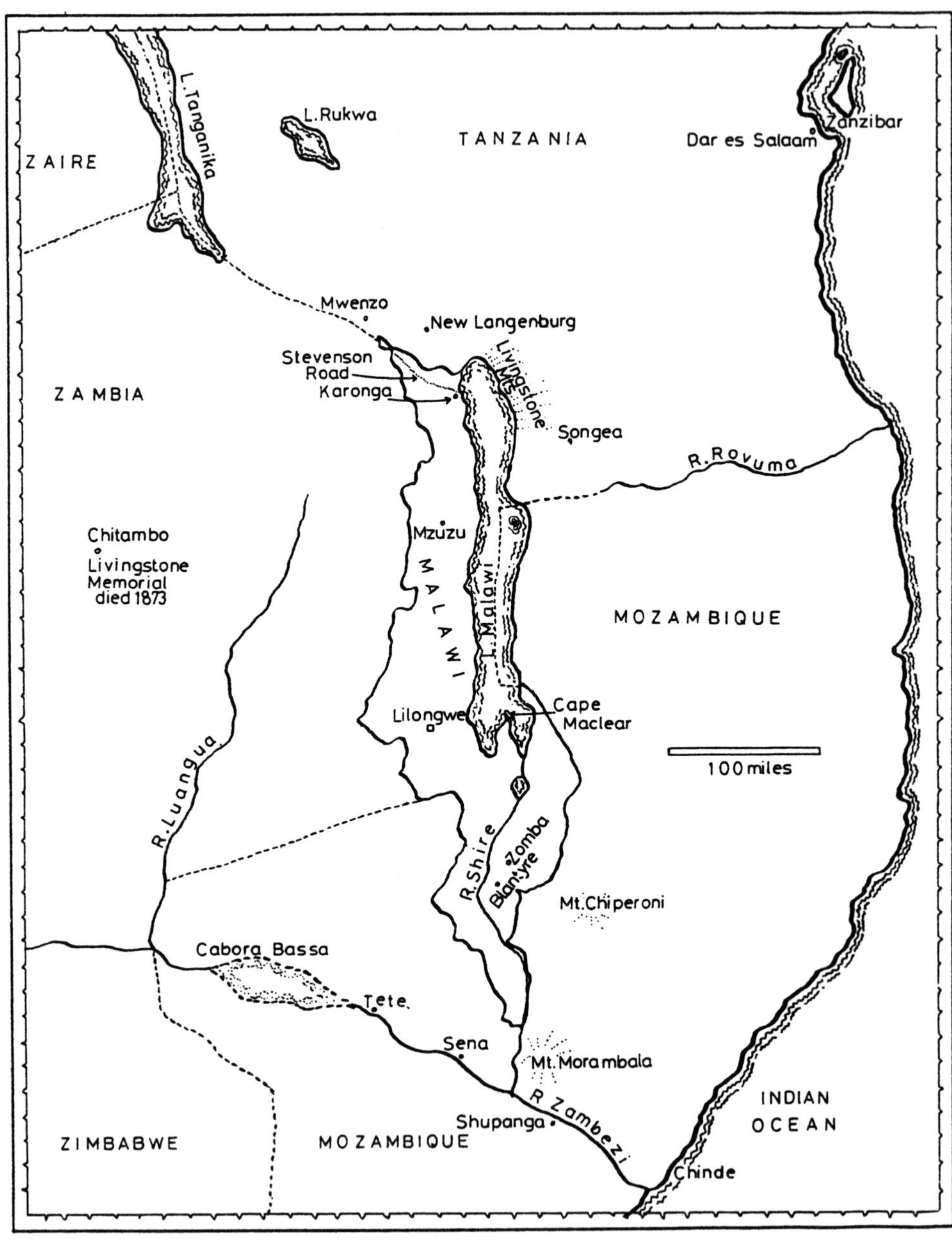
ZAIRE
ZAMBIA
TANZANIA
Dar es Salaam
Zanzibar
L.Tanganika
L.Rukwa
Mwenzo
New Langenburg
Stevenson Road
Karonga
Livingstone
Songea
R.Rovuma
Chitambo
Livingstone Memorial died 1873
Mzuzu
MALAWI
L.Malawi
MOZAMBIQUE
R.Luangua
Lilongwe
Cape Maclear
100 miles
R.Shire
Zomba
Blantyre
Mt.Chiperoni
Cabora Bassa
Tete
Sena
Mt.Morambala
R.Zambezi
Shupanga
INDIAN OCEAN
ZIMBABWE
MOZAMBIQUE
Chinde

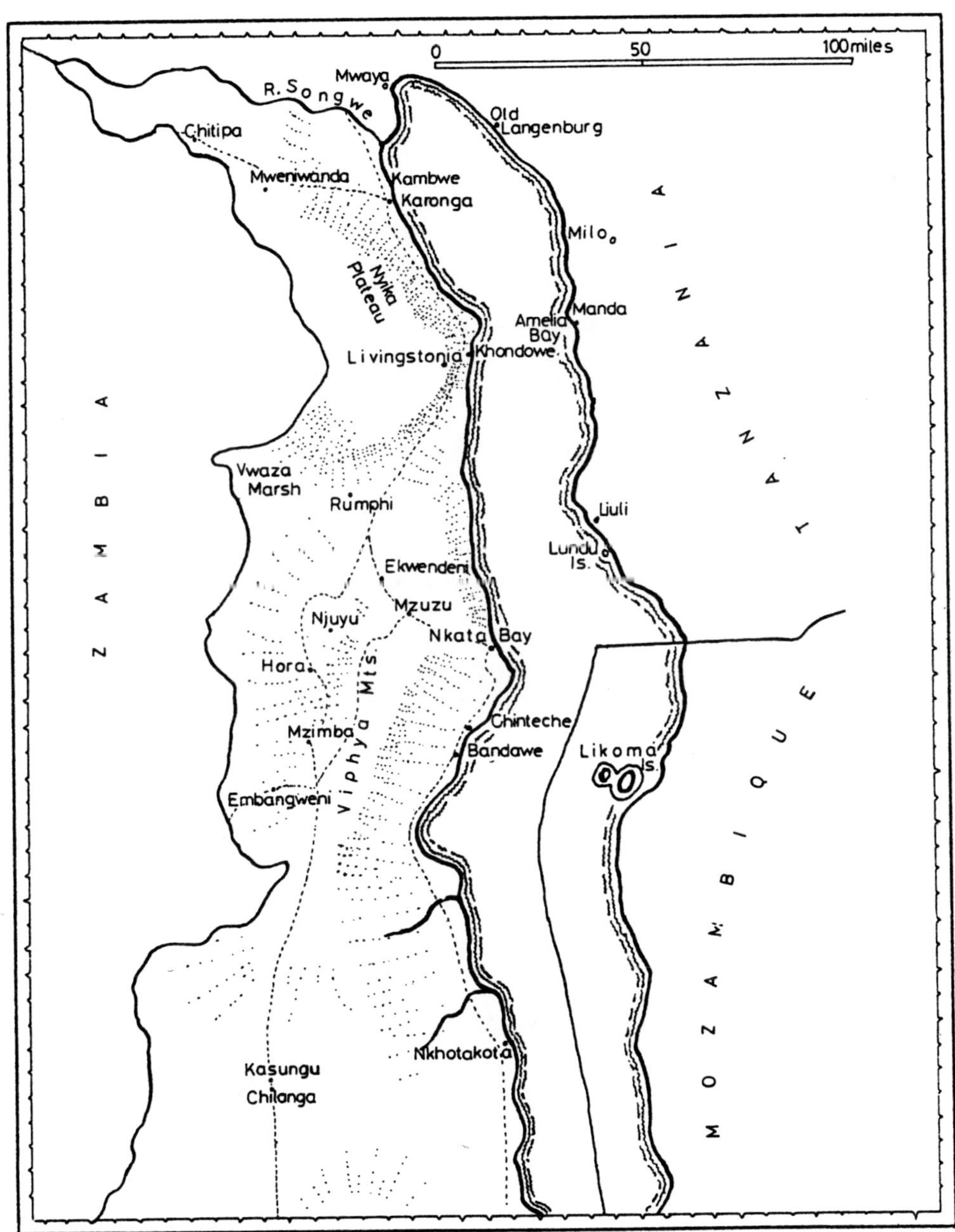

100 miles
50
0
Mwaya
R. Songwe
Old Langenburg
Chitipa
Mweniwanda
Kambwe
Karonga
Milo
Nyika Plateau
Manda
Amelia Bay
Livingstonia
Khondowe
ZAMBIA
TANZANIA
Vwaza Marsh
Rumphi
Liuli
Lundu Is.
Ekwendeni
Mzuzu
Njuyu
Nkata Bay
Hora
Viphya Mts
Chinteche
Mzimba
Bandawe
Likoma Is.
Embangweni
MOZAMBIQUE
Nkhotakota
Kasungu
Chilanga

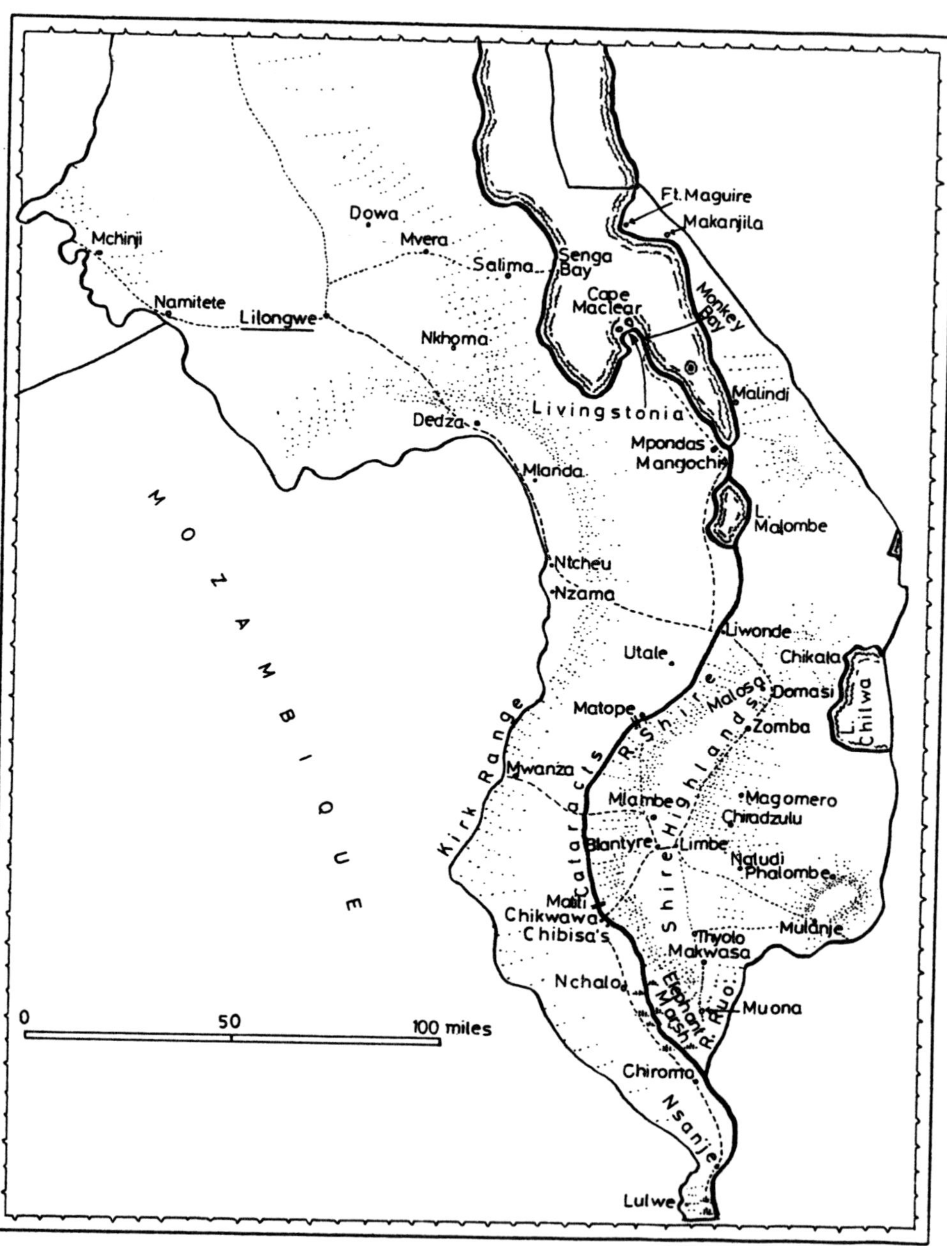

Ft. Maguire
Makanjila
Dowa
Mvera
Mchinji
Senga Bay
Salima
Cape Maclear
Monkey Bay
Namitete
Lilongwe
Nkhoma
Malindi
Livingstonia
Dedza
Mpondas
Mangochi
Mlanda
L. Malombe
MOZAMBIQUE
Ntcheu
Nzama
Liwonde
Utale
Chikala
R. Shire
Maloso
Domasi
Matope
Zomba
L. Chilwa
Kirk Range
Shire Highlands
Mwanza
Mlambe
Magomero
Chiradzulu
Blantyre
Limbe
Cataracts
Ngludi
Phalombe
Matiti
Chikwawa
Muljnje
Chibisa's
Thyolo
Makwasa
Nchalo
Elephant Marsh
R. Ruo
Muona
Chiroma
Nsanje
Lulwe
0   50   100 miles

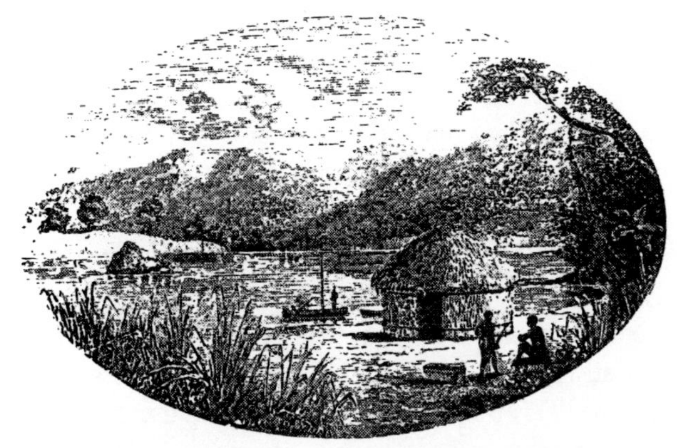

Camp at Matiti, near the Murchison Cataracts.

INTRODUCTION

June 9th 1863, at Matiti, where the Mwambezi Stream enters the Shire River, at the foot of the Cataracts:

"Fleeing for their lives and hotly pursued, they reached the river bank about a cables' length ahead of our vessel, and plunged into the river. The woman in question, less fortunate than others, was struck down by an arrow as she rose to the surface. Entering just below the left shoulder blade, the cruelly barbed head passed into her lungs; and when Dr.Livingstone, Dr.Kirk, and Dr.Meller, saw her a few hours afterwards, it was decided by the council of surgeons that the attempt to extricate it would only add to her terrible sufferings, and cause her a more speedy death. Extraordinary to relate, the men of the village took upon themselves to do that which no one better versed in such matters dare justify for a minute. Fastening a piece of string to the iron head, they drew it back by main force, cutting off the entangled flesh from the large fang-like barbs, and actually repeating the same process as portions of the lung appeared! Our astonishment was complete the next day to find no fatal symptoms had set in. Each day I saw to her diet myself. She now came forward (twelve years later in 1875) to greet us, bringing me a present of a fowl, and from all appearances had shaken off the ill effects of a barbarous operation in every sense of the word." (E.D.Young R.N. "Nyasa: A Journal of Adventures" 1877)

This is one of the first accounts of the meeting of Western and Traditional medicine in what is now Malaŵi. European medicine at that time had a restricted range. The early doctors, all missionaries, came from Britain at a time when important discoveries were about to be made. Anaesthesia was only a few years old, and antiseptic surgery had just been described. The link between bacteria and infection, and between malaria and mosquitoes, was to be proven in the future. There were few effective drugs of any sort.

Early on Africans were trained as dressers in wound treatment for outpatients. Government doctors were later appointed by the administration mainly to treat its employees, and to institute public health measures. By 1911, there were 29 doctors, many of whom left for the war effort in 1914.

In subsequent decades the country's health was improved by greater understanding of disease, more effective treatment, and public health measures. Most benefit was felt by the Government employees and those near Missions. The majority of the people would still rely on the herbalist and witchdoctor, and regard illness as something to be borne stoically, an attitude still prevalent today in rural areas.

After the Second World War, the coming of antibiotics and insecticides gave potent weapons to health workers. Many new hospitals and dispensaries were set up to attend the increasing population. Maternal and child health services spread. The numbers of local medical assistants and nurses increased, and the first Malawian doctors qualified abroad. In 1991 the Malawi College of Medicine opened.

Disease patterns have changed over this short period of 130 years. Feared diseases like smallpox and yaws, have gone, and leprosy is decreasing. However tuberculosis is increasing its hold, and a new disease, Aids, has appeared.

There are many factors involved in the prevalence and impact of disease on a country. One is the effort of the health workers to understand and improve the health climate. This is the story of a continuing effort in the lifetime of a nation.

1   BEFORE LIVINGSTONE

The original inhabitants of present day Malaŵi were hunter gatherer Bushmen. Around 1300 A.D. the Bantu tribal migrations were spreading southwards down from West Africa.These people kept animals, grew crops, and worked iron. They probably painted the white animal figures found in some rock shelters, just as the Bushmen are thought to have painted the red geometric figures. The Bantu tribes gradually split up into different groups and were known as Maravi by the early Portuguese. The Portuguese established forts along the East African coast at the end of the 15th Century, and later had trading posts up the Zambesi River, as far as Tete.

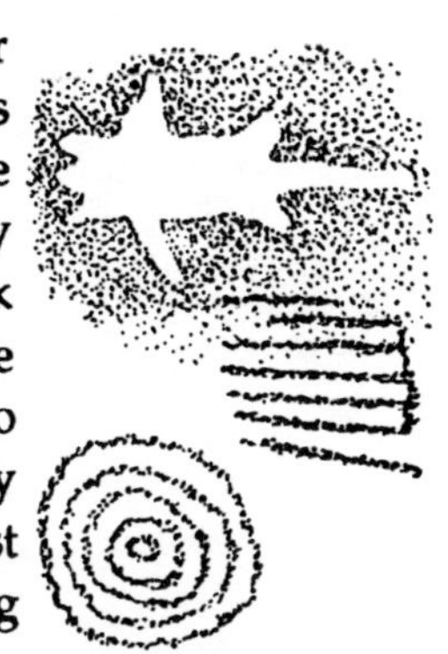

In the first half of the 19th century there were several migrations into Malaŵi. The East Coast Arabs and Afro/Arabs set up trading and slave posts around Lake Nyasa. The Yao tribes from the East Coast entered the country, and many were converted to Islam. The Ngoni, a warlike Zulu tribe, migrated up through the country, and then returned and settled in the North and Central highlands.

This was the time of the slave trade, and in some years as many as 30,000 slaves crossed the Lake in dhows on their journey to the coast. Tribes were set against tribes to capture slaves. It was into these many conflicts that Livingstone and the early missionaries came.

David Livingstone at the age of 42, had crossed Southern Africa in the years 1853-6. With him were his Makololo carriers who came from the Chobe Zambesi region above the Victoria Falls. The final part of the way he travelled down the Zambesi, left his carriers at Tete and returned to England. He was determined to do something about the Slave Trade, which he called "this open sore of Africa", and to bring enlightenment to the region.

In a famous speech at the Senate House in Cambridge in 1857, he said "I go back to Africa to make an open path for commerce and Christianity. Do you carry on the work I have begun? I leave it to you." As a result, the Universities' Mission to Central Africa (Cambridge, Oxford, Durham, and Dublin,) was founded. The next year, with British Government support, he travelled up the Zambesi in the *Ma-Robert*, collecting his Makololo carriers. Finding the impassable barrier of the Kebrabassa Rapids, he returned downstream, and ascended the Shire River (pronounced Shirree). Walking overland with

Dr.Kirk around the Shire Cataracts, they reached Lake Nyasa (now Lake Malaŵi) in September 1859.

In 1861, Livingstone in the *Pioneer* (*Ma-Robert's* replacement) collected the U.M.C.A. missionaries, headed by Bishop Mackenzie, at the Zambesi mouth and took them up the Shire River. On board were three doctors, Livingstone, Kirk, and Meller.

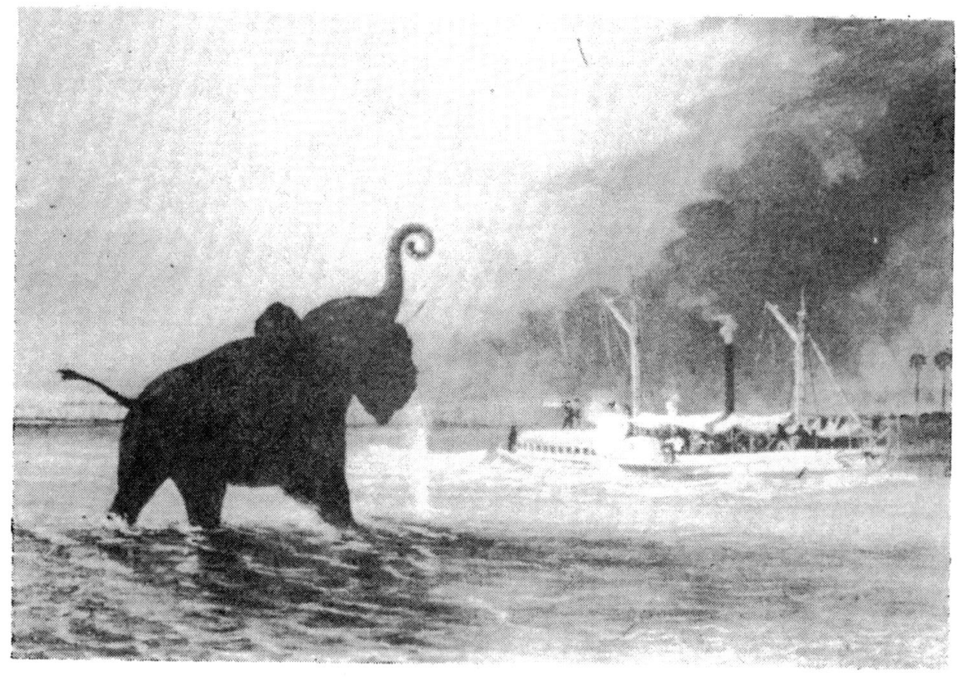

Ma Robert in the Elephant Marsh

2 THE ZAMBESI EXPEDITION

DR. DAVID LIVINGSTONE (served 1859-63)

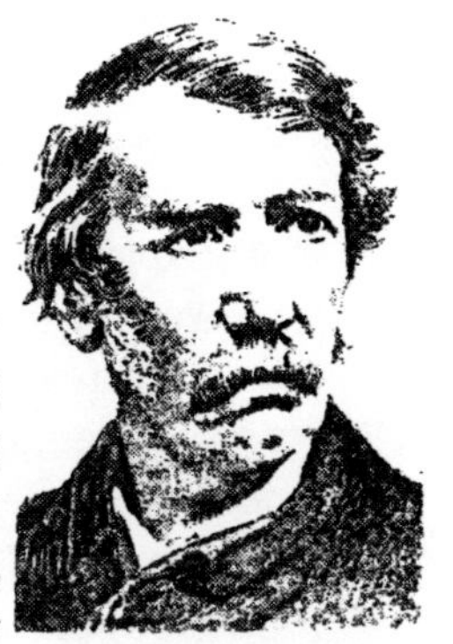

Dr. Livingstone

David Livingstone's Zambesi Expedition, which included the Universities' Mission of Oxford, Cambridge, Durham, and Dublin, opened the door to modern medicine and brought four outstanding doctors to the Shire River.

On January 1st 1859, Dr.Livingstone and Dr.Kirk steamed up the Shire in the **Ma-Robert**...."we met many people coming down in canoes, we passed many fishing boats moored by strong ropes, we see many traps for killing hippopotami. We now take our quinine again...villages very numerous, and cassava, rice, beans, tobacco, pumpkins, ochra, and millet, grow luxuriantly. Saw several herds of elephants, at one time a hundred were in sight." Within a week they reached present day Chikwawa, where they were welcomed by Chief Chibisa, whom Livingstone described as "a jolly person who laughs easily; he lives on a river bank 100 feet high and nearly perpendicular. I explained that we made observations of the stars using instruments, for the purpose of laying down paths for our friends, and he must not think of witchcraft. He replied that we were not to be alarmed by the singing of his people." Chief Chibisa's Village became the sanctuary of this expedition.

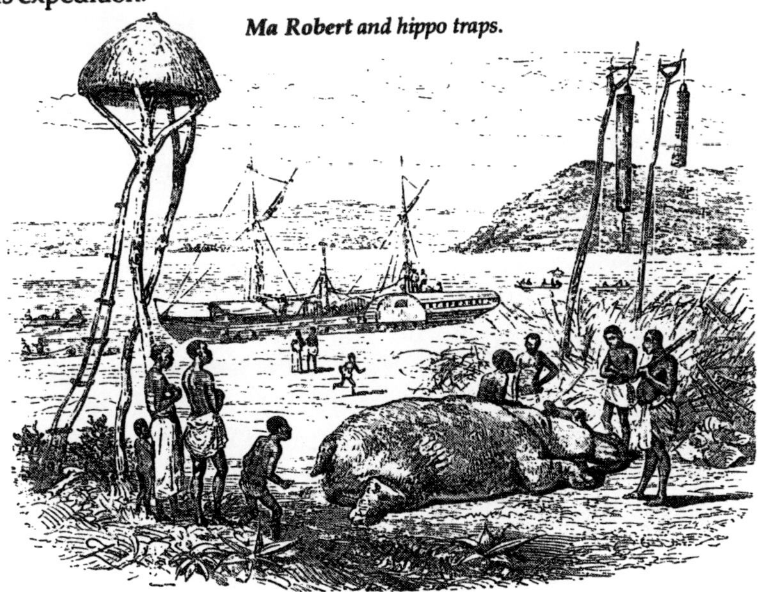

Ma Robert and hippo traps.

David Livingstone had been taught at Glasgow Medical School to make objective scientific judgements based on personal observation. As previous attempts to explore the Zambesi had been defeated by malaria, he regarded quinine as the essential prophylactic. He wrote in his Zambesi Report "Quinine was taken by all Europeans with a single exception, to the amount of two grains in sherry every day. Our own experience in the highlands between the Shire River and Lake Chilwa during 24 days ... over rough country, under the tropical sun, and sleeping in the open air, was to enjoy perfect health, as did the Africans who were with us." He saw that the cinchona tree producing quinine grew in abundance at Sena, close to modern Nsanje, and "where the fever prevails, there the remedy abounds." His observations of disease in the local African people are interesting. He commented that while pneumonia was common, TB did not occur at all then in the African population. He noticed that disease epidemics occur in the rainy season.

He was aware of the psychological value of African tradition. He described a funeral dance at Chibisa's village: "we found two circles of people dancing, with drums and wailing. Four drums were beaten and medicines were burned. An old woman with calabashes in her hands danced with tears streaming down her cheeks, and the mother of the dead child was taken away in a faint."

In October 1859, after a long journey on foot with Kirk, Dr. Livingstone wrote about his own health: "very ill with bleeding from bowels and purging. Bled all night. We have all had touches of illness. 300 miles in the hottest season of the year is too much for Europeans without English food..." The coming of the mango season enabled him to recover by December. "Mangoes ripe at present; freely used they seem to excite kidneys and bowels, and preserve health."

Livingstone departed to the Zambesi in December 1859 and returned to the Shire River in July 1861 with the Universities Mission led by Bishop Mackenzie. He escorted them to settle at Magomero, which is to the southeast of the modern Blantyre to Zomba road. Here he noticed a high incidence of leprosy. On his voyage along the west coast of Lake Nyasa in September 1861, he observed many skin diseases in the Salima area, including leprosy. He also noted a case of elephantiasis, caused by filarial worms, at Kabango Bay, near Nkhota Kota. On a huge shady tree by St. Anne's Church Nkhota Kota is an inscription: "In memory of Dr. Livingstone's arrival at Nkhota Kota in 1861. He rested at the foot of this tree where he met Jumbe and other

Chewa Chiefs and made a treaty with them."

Livingstone is credited with being the first doctor to have noticed that an insect bite causes disease. He suggested that relapsing fever is caused by a tick bite. He commented favourably on the absence of tsetse flies in the Shire Highlands. He gave the first description of the boil produced by the maggot fly here: "a small tumour formed on Wilson's shoulder, and Dr.Kirk having touched it with nitrate of silver, a grub like minute bot was taken out. Jumbo subsequently took one out of his thigh, and Wilson from his ankle."

Records survive of five of his patients here: A little Ajawa girl named Chasika "had always been a special favourite with Dr. Livingstone during two years of great suffering she underwent from acute disease at Magomero." She had an ulcer of her foot and was unable to walk, and later married Chinsoro, freed from a slave caravan (Young 1867); Endamoschule covered with leprosy at Matiti; "The woman shot by the Ajawa with an arrow is recovering. It was cut out by the people themselves"; "Moloka is ill again with a fresh abscess"; "The wound inflicted on Longe is healing. It went in slanting and though his lungs are a little affected, he is well".

David Livingstone was the last member of the Zambesi Expedition to leave in 1863, after several had died of malaria. On his last journey down the Shire River, he passed the graves of Richard Thornton at Kapachira Falls, of Dickinson and Scudamore at Chibisa's Village, of Ferger in the Elephant Marsh, of Bishop Mackenzie at Chiromo, and of his beloved wife Mary, at Shupunga. He was not defeated by these disasters. The problems of the local people who were beset by a brutal slave trade, by tribal conflicts, by starvation, and by disease, strengthened his determination to help them.

DR. JOHN KIRK Surgeon/Botanist (served 1859-63)

John Kirk was 26 years old when he accompanied the veteran Dr.Livingstone on his first journey up the Shire River. He had qualified in a distinguished class at the Edinburgh Royal Infirmary, which included Joseph Lister, the founder of antiseptic surgery. He was appointed to the Zambesi Expedition to collect plants for Kew Gardens. He was an expert botanist and pioneer photographer. He took the first photographs in the country.

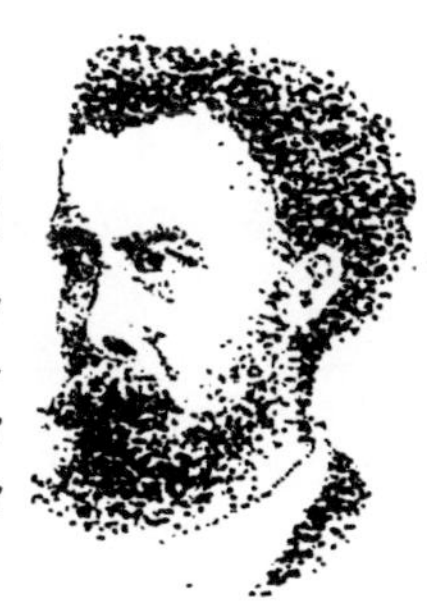

Dr. Kirk

On arrival at Chibisa's Village in 1859, Livingstone wrote "Kirk

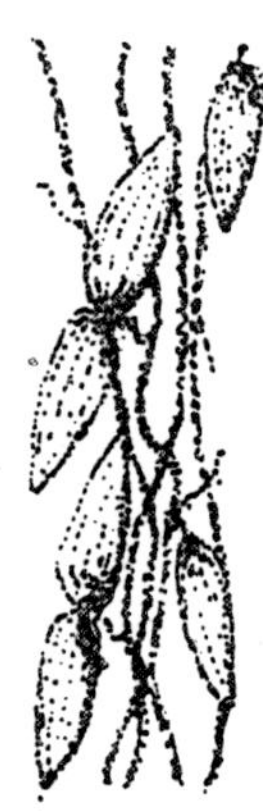

Kombe

got the poison, Kombe, which they use for their arrows. It is seen in abundance about the river. It is a climber and has pods about 14 inches long united end to end." Later,"Dr.Kirk found a true floating sensitive plant on the river."

On September 17th 1859, Kirk and Livingstone having walked 150 miles up the east bank of the Shire River, reached Lake Nyasa at present day Mangochi. It was called Lake Ninyessi, or Lake of the Stars. They were the first Europeans to see "this splendid Lake, cranes, reeds on the bank, two islands visible, mountains on either side." Sadly, in this area, Kirk first saw a gang of Arab slavers on the march, laden with ivory, malachite, and copper. Their Arab captors offered to sell him some children, but "on understanding we were English made off during the night, although they must have been a hundred strong with guns among them. The slaves were forced on by a long pole, forked at one end, in which the slaves's neck was fastened, while the other was carried on the man's shoulder behind. At night the free end was fastened to a tree."

Next day they met more parties of slavers, one party who again offered slaves for sale was going east, a second Swahili party was coming up from the coast and trading in malachite. Encounters like this were continual, and clearly dozens of slave gangs were daily driving hundreds of slaves across this country. John Kirk gallantly attacked numerous slave drivers himself and freed the helpless people who were their victims, including many

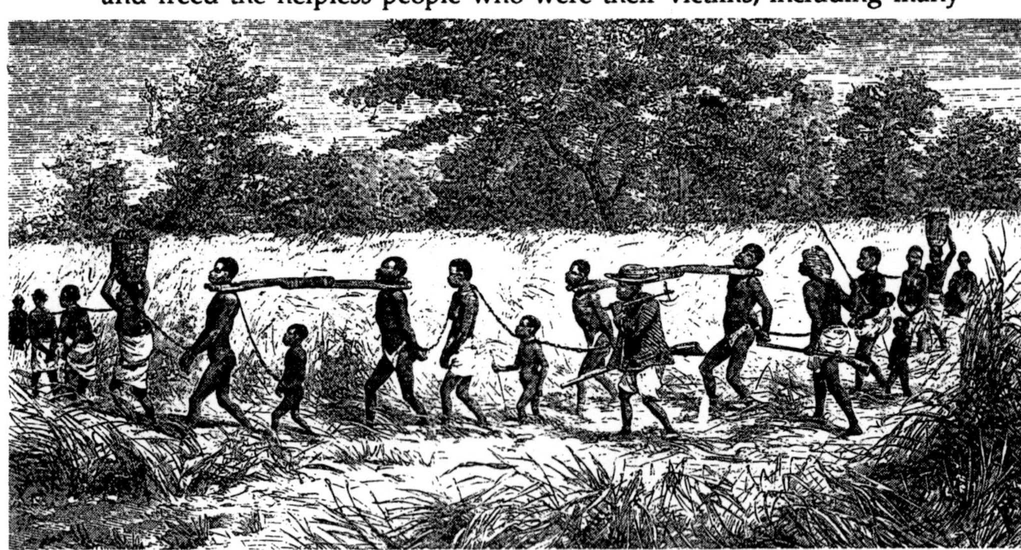

Slave Caravans (after a drawing by Livingstone).

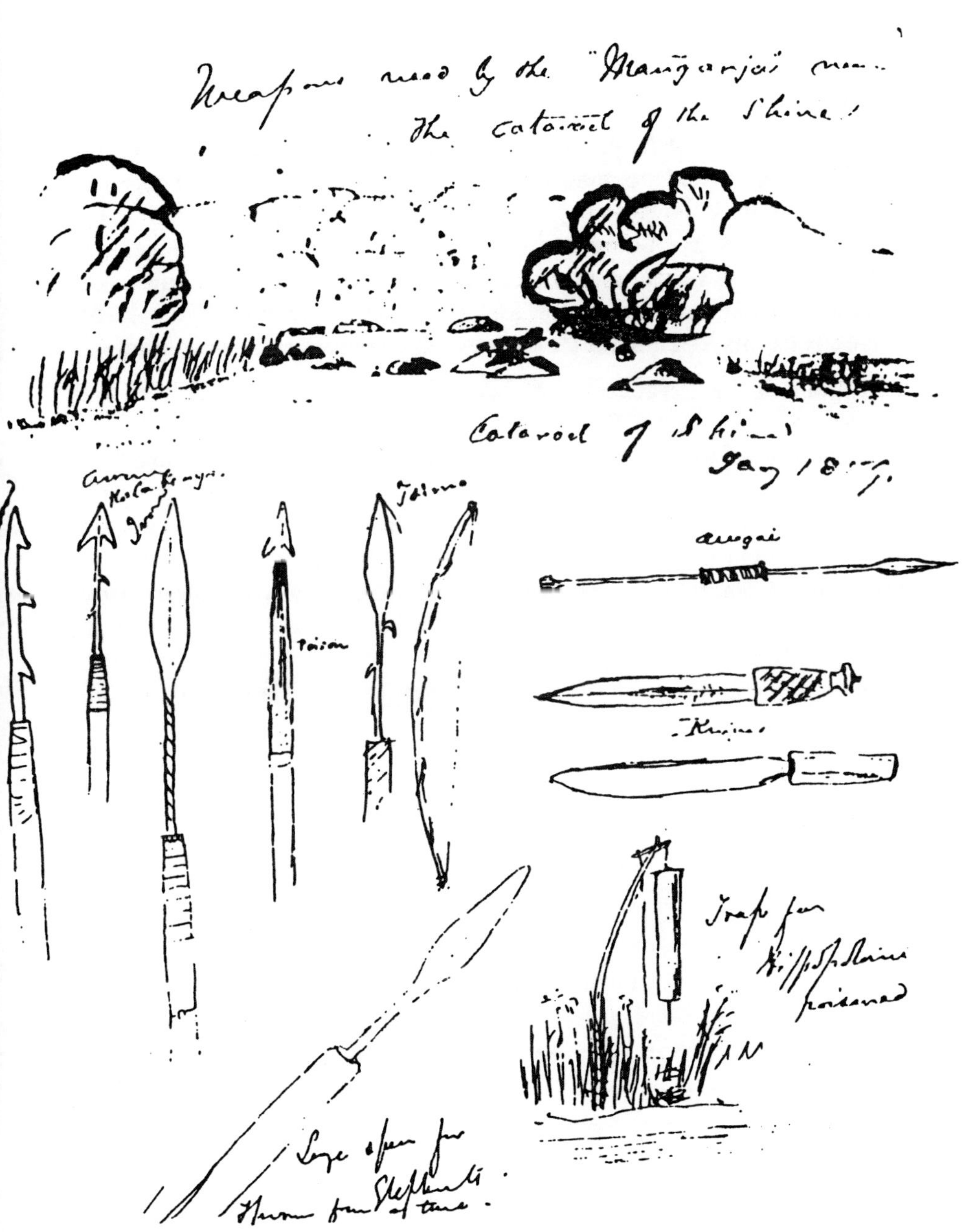

From Kirk's sketch book Jan. 1859

women and children. He realised the more terrible consequences of this slave trade; the slavers often paid chiefs of one tribe to capture slaves from another, so tribal conflicts were instigated. The Yaos were attacking the Chewas for this reason.

Kirk's scientific curiosity enabled him to write the first clinical description of Blackwater Fever. Until then it had been confused with Yellow Fever. On his voyage with Livingstone up the west coast of Lake Nyasa in 1861, Kirk noted in the vicinity of modern Salima "The people are ill-nourished and sickly, disease is frequent; we see many cases of leprosy and other skin diseases, diseases of the eye, club foot, and other deformities of the limbs. Smallpox has marked many." He commented on the high infant death rate.

Dr.Kirk made the first collection of fishes and reptiles from Lake Nyasa and the Shire River. Mr.A.Gunther reported on Kirk's findings in the "Proceedings of the Zoological Society" of London in 1864. He noted the great variety of endemic Cichlid species. He also reported mammals: "On the western shore of Lake Nyasa, on a rocky headland which ran out into the Lake, we saw a number of Black Monkeys quite different from any met elsewhere. No specimens were obtained as the boat was moving quickly, and heavy seas were running at the time." John Kirk himself began to succumb to the harsh environment, "in fact, 250 miles in this season (September 1861), and in this country on foot, and with strange food, is enough for the strongest."

Dr.Kirk attended both Dr.and Mrs.Livingstone. He knew of the doctor's fine ability to deal kindly with the local Africans - "If the Doctor keeps good health he can manage them, but if his digestive system don't go all right, he loses his diplomatic powers wonderfully."

When Livingstone left the Shire in 1863, Kirk wrote to him: "Do you intend to have your arm (injured by a lion) set right? Anything surgical go to Syme at Edinburgh, don't get into the hands of the London surgeons whatever you do."

Mrs.Livingstone died on April 27th 1862 at Shupunga on her intended journey to the Shire River. Kirk looked after her as she lay ill with malaria for two weeks in a tent beside the Zambesi. On April 27th he noted "Mrs.Livingstone became worse and worse, steadily coma deepened and the skin tinged of a deep yellow, and at 7 pm she died. We dug a deep grave under the baobab tree."

Livingstone attacked by a lion, 1843 in South Africa.

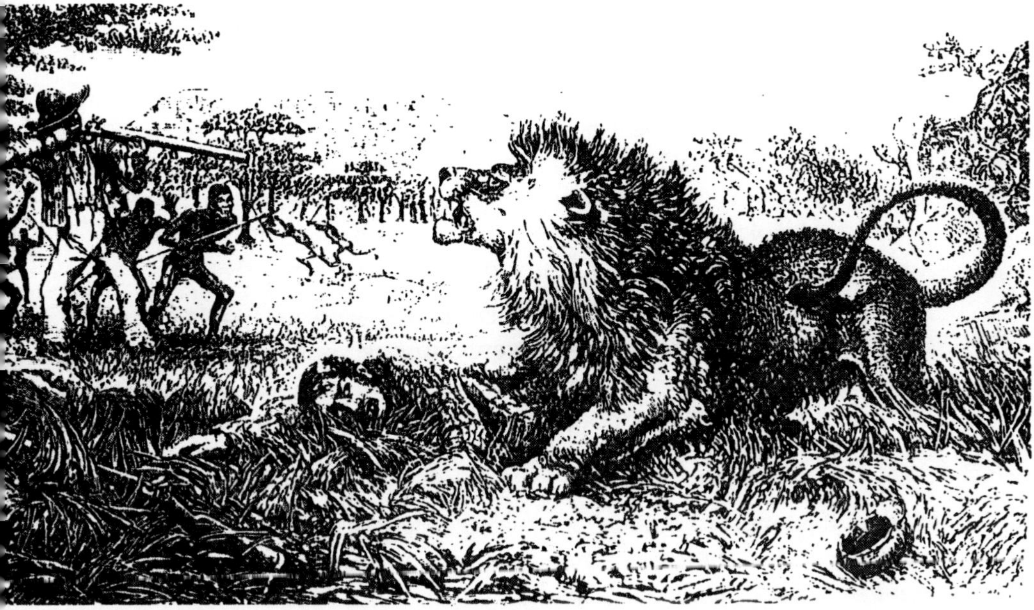

After five years sojourn by the Shire River, Kirk's inspiration was overwhelmingly humanitarian. Having seen the full extent and horror of the slave trade here, he devoted the rest of his long career as British consul at Zanzibar to a determined and successful campaign to stop the slave trade. Slavery disappeared from East Africa. Today, to the west of the M1 Blantyre to Balaka main road, lie the high mountains of the Kirk Range, named after him.

DR. CHARLES MELLER Surgeon/Naturalist (served 1859-63)

Charles Meller arrived in the Shire Valley in 1861 as ship's doctor to the *Pioneer*. When his boat anchored at Chibisa's Village, Meller went regularly up to the Zomba plain to visit the Mission at Magomero. Bishop Mackenzie wrote of the difficulties the missionaries faced in the tribal wars and slave trade at Magomero:

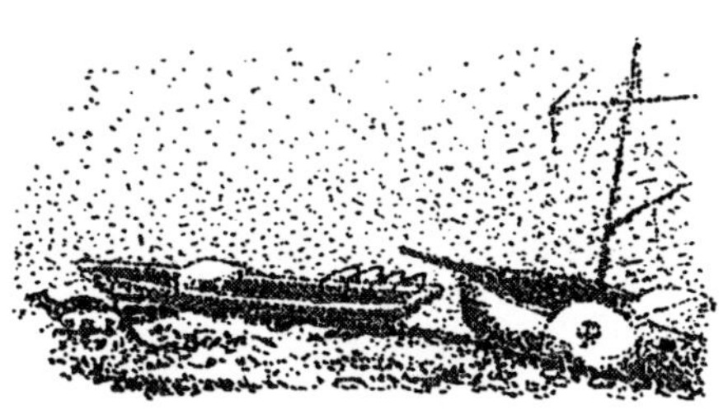

Lady Nyassa alongside the Pioneer (from a photo by Kirk.)

"October 17th 1861 - We got away at 6 a.m. as loading more than 30 Manganja guns took more than an hour I suppose. Dr. Meller would be called in England quite unfit for anything. Two others of our party were quite unwell."

There Meller made an early record of a surgical patient in Malaŵi: "one poor fellow had such a heel as I never saw. He was struck in it by accident with a fish spear; the whole tendon is gone and the bone decaying beneath. In this state he was driven 30 miles by the slavers and came back 40 with us. he never complains." Sadly, the terrible wounds inflicted on slaves then kept Dr.Meller busy. However he found time to make many sketches.*

Meller did the first disease survey in Central Africa, on malaria. His findings "On Fever of East Central Africa" were published in the "British Medical Journal" in 1862, and in the "Lancet" in 1864. He made a careful comparison of this disease in different groups of people in the Zambesi Expedition (see the chapter on malaria), concluding that the local Africans "have an almost perfect immunity to malaria" which the visitors lacked. His pioneer observations are still of value today - the concept of malarial immunity, and his descriptions of different manifestations of malaria such as dysentery, vomiting, blackwater fever, cerebral malaria with fits, mania, or mental disorder.

Meller recommended full doses of quinine at the onset of malaria. Forty years before it was known that malaria was transmitted by mosquitoes, Meller advised people to avoid being bitten by mosquitoes and to care for their general health, as important prophylactic measures. "Ensure a dry sleeping place and warm clothing at night. A good mosquito net for the bed should be provided. Each person should drink hot coffee on rising and eat a mixed diet."

Dr.Meller devotedly cared for his patients. He was very distressed by the death in 1863 of young Richard Thornton, geologist to the Zambesi Expedition. "During 1858-62 in Africa he had very good health and no fever. He was accustomed to travel in his own boat (canoe), sleeping anywhere and roughing it in all weathers. He abjured medicine altogether, and had not taken quinine since coming into this country. In March 1863, he undertook a walk of 150 miles to fetch supplies, and returned much exhausted after walking through miles of rank high grass. A week later he was seized with fever....diarrhoea, vomiting, mania, coma.....quinine was vomited...after 11 days he died at Matiti". (On the west bank of the Shire River near the Cataracts, his grave is under a baobab tree). Livingstone

* Illus. p.97.

wrote "Dr.Meller got into a mortal funk on poor Thornton's death, and went around telling each of the men that unless invalided at once, he would not be responsible for his life."

In July 1863, Dr.Meller departed, travelling down the Shire River in a dugout canoe. He himself became very ill with cerebral malaria after a night on a mud-flat in the Zambesi River, but survived. He was later Vice Consul in Madagascar, and died in Australia.

DR. JOHN DICKINSON (served 1861-63)

John Dickinson, the first resident doctor in this country, was a pioneer and prize-winning graduate of Newcastle Medical School. Owing to poor health, he was advised to go to Africa for sunshine! The Universities Mission found him superior to any other candidate, and he was appointed surgeon attached to Magomero Mission Station for a term of at least three years.

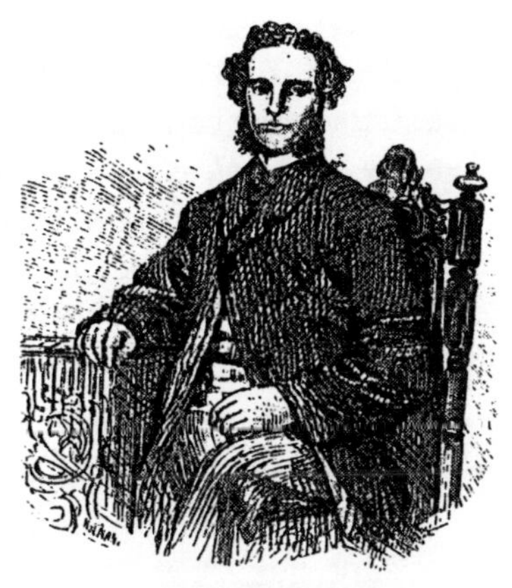

Dr. John Dickinson

Waller wrote of his arrival on the Shire River: "On November 29th 1861, at Chibisa's Village, while chatting away at breakfast, we heard two guns fired which assured us of the coming of Dr.Dickinson and Clark. I was quickly across the river, when a hearty 'All right Sir' from Charles, and the sight of two new faces told me our hopes and fears for their safety might now be cast to the winds. My hurrah now joined with others that came to welcome them."

Houses of mud and straw were being constructed at Magomero, but the Mission was beset with difficulties. Procuring food was the major problem. Rowley recorded "our people were starving. We did all we could to get food from the surrounding villages, going fifty miles from home to get it, but we could not procure enough. Our reserve stock was exhausted...and on Christmas Eve 1861 I distributed all the corn I had, there was not half a ration each. Dickinson had plenty of patients at this time. Many old ulcers had been cured, but many were incurable, and new ones were continually breaking out. The dormitory for the boys was turned into a hospital, and Dickinson's zeal never flagged, his charity never failed."

Dickinson advised the Mission to leave Magomero because it was an

	From Dr. Dickinson's records.		
Name	**Date**	**Disease**	**Duration**
Proctor	6th	fever	3 days
Proctor	26th	fever	6 days
Scudamore	11th	fever	6 days
Rowley	20th	neuralgia	2 days
Dickinson	26th	fever	5 days

unhealthy situation, and on May 6th 1862, the missionaries returned to Chibisa's Village by the Shire River. Here though, the dangers of malaria were worse. He kept careful notes on his patients at Chibisa's. In June 1862 eleven missionaries were ill with fever.

On August 2nd 1862, James Stewart visited this Mission at Chibisa's Village, and wrote "saw round the Station, the dining hall, chapel, huts, stone huts and surgery. The huts are small, though large enough for one man, round, and tolerably comfortable...there are 112 Africans in the care of the Mission, some have left, as many as 50 have died of ulcers and other causes. Bananas are still plentifully cultivated.....soon I was introduced to Proctor, Rowley, and Dickinson. Poor Dickinson's face and appearance were a sad comment on the unhealthiness of the district. His bloodless face and intense weakness were touching indeed. He had fever and haematuria."

John Dickinson trained the first medical dresser in Malaŵi. Captain E.D.Young wrote in 1867 that a boy named Sinjeri was liberated from slavers by Livingstone and Mackenzie, and became assistant to Dr.Dickinson in his pristine surgery at Chibisa's Village. "I remember the amusement he had in helping Dr. Dickinson's microscopical studies. One day the search was for diatoms (microscopic life), master and boy might be seen taking alternate squints down the tube of the microscope at diatomy looking weed". On August 14th, Dr.Dickinson took into his care Chief Muloka, who had received eight wounds when charged by an elephant at nearby Mankokwi's Village, and was brought by canoe upstream to Chibisa's. He nursed him to recovery.

Then the summer rains failed, and a terrible famine hit the Shire Valley. More than half the population died of starvation. The Mission stated "wild looking men, worn almost to skeletons, with cords tied around their waists to lessen the pangs of hunger, roamed around, grubbing up roots, until unable to go on any longer they sank down and died."

On November 6th 1862, Stewart wrote in his diary "news from Chibisa's: great scarcity of food; crocodile carried off Mashiho's wife; Proctor and Scudamore ill with severe dysentery, Rowley and Dickinson with ulcerous sores on the hands which refuse to heal."

Dickinson was unwilling to leave the Shire until another doctor came to replace him. In his spare time he made a natural history collection and spent hours bird watching in the marshes of the Shire River. His ornithological

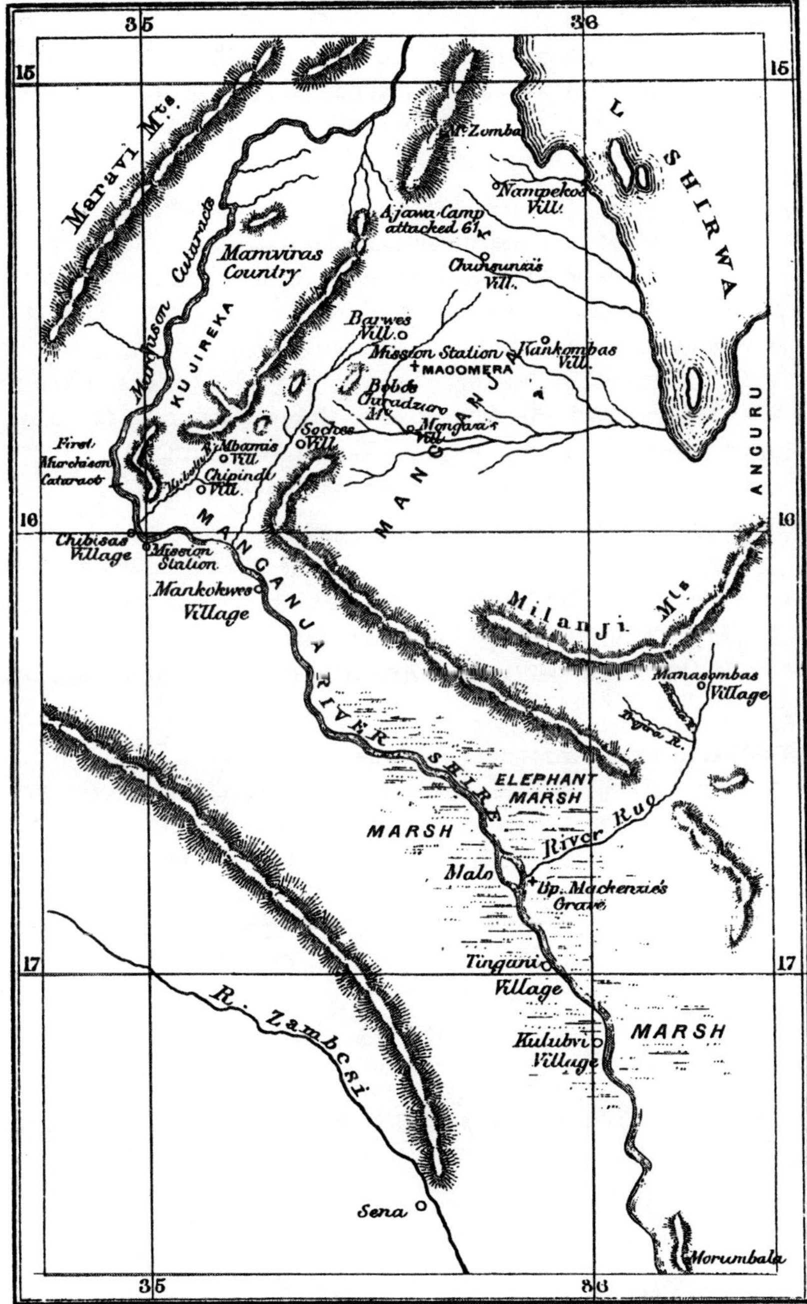

RIVER SHIRE, & COUNTRY OCCUPIED BY THE MISSION.

1867 Map

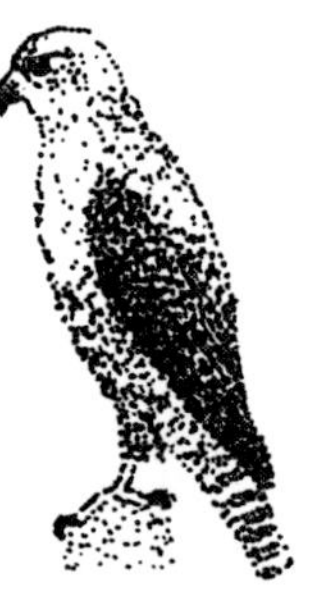

Dickinson's Falcon

collection consisted of 118 birds including 48 birds of prey. The most important of these was a falcon, previously unknown, which was later named "Falco Dickinsoni". He also made a considerable collection of diatomaceae.

On Christmas Day 1862 Rowley wrote "Scudamore was not better. The fever seemed less violent, but his tongue and his throat were much ulcerated and an abscess was forming dangerously near the larynx. Dickinson had a fever which made him totter, but nothing could exceed his kind and incessant attention to Scudamore for whom he had a great regard." In January 1863 Dickinson recorded Scudamore's death "from inflammation of the parotid gland, neck, and breast. This was of an erysipelatous form and was difficult of treatment from the state of weakness to which he was reduced by fever."

On March 17th 1863 "dear devoted Dickinson, after a severe illness of eight days, has died." Livingstone and Kirk had been called from the *Pioneer* to his assistance, but arrived half an hour too late. He was buried beside Scudamore at Chibisa's Village. The graves are to the south of the modern Blantyre to Chikwawa road, on the west bank of the Shire River close to the bridge.

In 1876 Young wrote "we paid a visit to the graves of Henry Scudamore and John Dickinson at Chibisa's Village, only to find the same deep respect evinced for their preservation. Future generations will come to hear of these men who wrenched the slave sticks from their fathers and mothers, and who endured the hard days of famine and destruction with them". Chief Muloka named his son "Dickinson". Newcastle Medical School still awards an annual Prize in memory of the work in Malaŵi of John Dickinson.

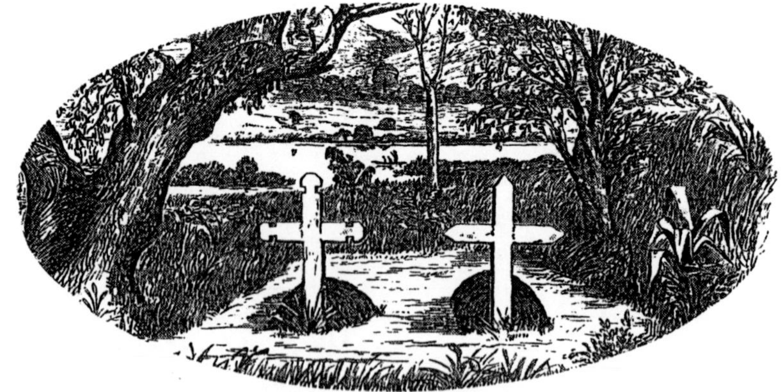

Scudamore and Dickinson's Graves

3 MALARIA

"One day's fever takes away the health of the whole year" Swahili proverb

19 Zambesimen	none dead		1% of time sick
10 Johannamen (Comoros)	none dead		3% of time sick
10 Europeans	4 died,	3 invalided home,	20% of time sick

These are Dr.Meller's observations on the Zambesi and Shire expeditions in 1859. It illustrates the severe effects of malaria on visitors and the lesser effects on locals, because of their immunity. "Burrup is very low and we have run out of quinine which we ought to be taking every day, there is none." Bishop Mackenzie died from want of the lost quinine in 1861, the first of the long list of Europeans who died of malaria in the country. Livingstone recognized the value

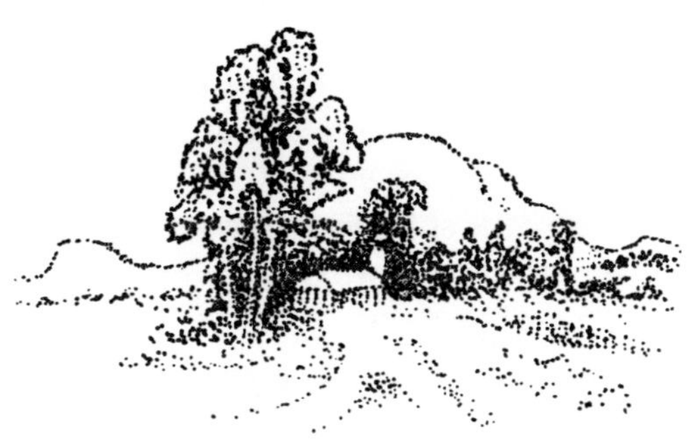

Magomero today with a memorial chapel near the grave of Rev. Burrup who died of malaria in 1862

of quinine, which had been used for fevers since the 17th century, as Jesuit, or Peruvian bark from the cinchona tree. He had noted its protection in Dr.M'William's account of the Niger Expedition of 1842. Livingstone devised his pill or 'Rouser' containing quinine and a purgative and dosed a patient

Extract from the Lancet 1862

"until the ears ring" (deafness and noises in the ears are side effects). Later he used it as a preventative or prophylactic "two grains in sherry every day".

"The urine was from the first of a deep green colour subsequently going through shades of brown and black." This is Kirk's account of blackwater fever, a severe complication of malaria, when altered blood pigments are passed out in the urine. It is seen in non-immune patients and is related to the use of quinine. Kirk also carried out the first autopsy or post-mortem by the Shire River on Mr.Ferger, the carpenter of the *Pioneer*, who died of malaria in December 1861: "On examination the organs were all healthy except the spleen which was enlarged and quite soft, in fact almost fluid. It broke to pieces when lifted up."

The connection between fever, swamps, and bad air, (miasmata or mal'aria) had long been suspected. At Cape Maclear in 1876, after Dr.Laws had had 15 attacks of fever in a few months, they decided to drain the swamp behind the Mission by a gulley into the Lake. Miasmata was thought to be spread horizontally, so sleeping on platforms or in a two storey building was thought helpful. Even before the connection between mosquitoes and malaria was made, using mosquito nets and wearing high boots or two pairs of socks in the evening was advised.

The sickness and death rate among the first Europeans was high. It was a significant disease among Africans but at this stage there are only European figures. In 1887-88, 10% of Europeans died of fever (32 out of 300). On Likoma Island blackwater fever had a 33% mortality (12 deaths in 6 years). Dr.MacVicar* in Blantyre wrote in 1898 "Nearly every week some European dies of blackwater fever. The worst of it is that it is still so obscure a disease that one feels utterly helpless".

It was felt that those who recovered ran additional risks of recurrence and should probably leave the country. It was believed it was more common in the third year of residence, and so leave was advised after two years. One potent cause of blackwater fever was believed to be the release of "poison" on turning and digging the soil.

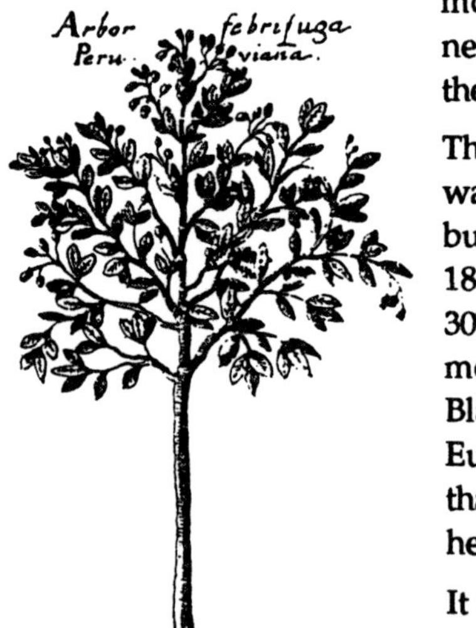

Fever bark tree from 1662 book.

Illus. inside front cover.

The treatment at that time was varied and idiosyncratic and consisted largely of nursing care. "What we would do without champagne I really do not know. They vomit everything else but champagne quiets the stomach and it is possible to get down small and frequent quantities of food." (W.Poole 1895). Mustard plasters were applied to loins and calves. Bleeding the patient was done. Wine, Liebeg's, Brand's Essence, Benger's Food, and Albert biscuits, were used to tempt the patient.

LIEBIG'S EXTRACT OF MEAT & MALT WINE
(COLEMAN'S),
A DELICIOUS BEVERAGE AND TONIC,

MADE from Port Wine, Liebig's Extract of Meat and Extract of Malt; Nutritious, Strengthening, Stimulating, Flesh-forming, and Health-restoring; suitable for the Robust in Health, as well as the Invalid. Strongly recommended by the Medical Faculty. An immediate Benefit is experienced after taking it; the Frame is Invigorated, and no ill effects follow.

The commanding officer of the Sikh soldiers, Lt.Col.Edwards*, was treated in Zomba for malaria by W.Poole in 1897: "Then he got blackwater fever, his temperature fell and it looked all right, but he had a rigor, then passed blackwater again. Every day he had a rigor, sometimes passed blackwater, sometimes being free, so that all his blood was drained away and it looked hopeless. Nothing did any good. I tried transfusions of blood from a native and the next day he was better and said: Well I think you've managed the job this time.' Then things went bad again. Often we thought he could not last; he was cold and clammy, with a pulse you could not count but he was wonderfully strong and got round. This went on for 20 days...then it became obvious he could not last more than a few hours. He was perfectly conscious until he died, made his will, arranged about his servants, said goodbye to us, saying he knew he had been selfish and then asked me if he would be long dying. We've never seen a man die so well."

That must have been the first blood transfusion in Malaŵi. It was probably done with a syringe or direct from the donor via a rubber tube. Quite likely the blood would have clotted, and it might have been just as well since blood groups were not then understood.

In 1896 Johnston wrote to the Foreign Office "I think we may once and for all get rid of the myth that British Central Africa has the slightest pretence to be any more healthy than any other place in Africa. What deceives us here is the

*Illus. inside back cover.

great beauty of the climate and the Shire Highlands." Two years later Dr.MacVicar and Fred Moir urged the Marquis of Salisbury to send a bacteriologist and equipment to Blantyre for blackwater fever research.

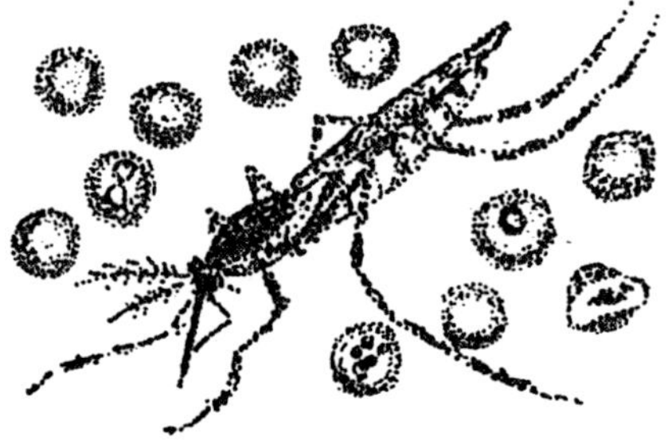

Anopheles mosquito. Magnified red blood cells comtaining malaria parasites.

At this time (1897 in India) Ronald Ross finally proved the connection between malaria and mosquitoes. He found the malarial organism in the mosquito. He wrote:

"I find thy cunning seeds
O, million murdering death."

Experts from the London School of Tropical Medicine came out to Blantyre Hospital and were given a ward for malaria research in 1899. The African Transcontinental Telegraph Company agreed that their services could be used free of charge to report cases of blackwater fever.

A greater awareness of the importance of not being bitten, drainage schemes, inspecting and clearing stagnant water, as well as improved buildings and the use of prophylactic quinine, reduced the morbidity (sickness) of malaria, at least in Blantyre. In 1897 a reliable injectable quinine (the bi-hydrochlorate) came into the country and this was very useful in vomiting patients.

"There was a habit to pile powdered quinine on a threepenny bit, wrap it up in cigarette paper and swallow it down with whisky which was cheap in those days." Others disagreed with the whisky and advocated abstinence. The African Lakes Company employed teetotallers: "in all my twenty years I have come across only two genuine teetotallers and I am sorry to say they both fill graves!" (Contemporary comment)

On Likoma Island, Dr.Howard experimented on himself,inducing deafness due to overdosage at one stage. He found that 15 grains a week was better than 5 grains a day for prophylaxis. However the incidence of malaria among the White Fathers was reduced when the Superior ordered five grains to be taken daily. The death rate although decreasing was still high, and of 133 missionaries between 1875-1915, 28 died and 10 were invalided home.

In 1906 the Railway Company building the line from Chiromo to Blantyre appointed a doctor for their 4,000 workers. He died within the year of blackwater fever in Luchenza. The type of malaria most common in Malaŵi is 'Falciparum'. It is also unfortunately the most serious of the four types.

Universities' Mission to Central Africa.

RULES OF HEALTH.

1. Take weekly doses of quinine: 10 grains on Monday night and 10 grains on Tuesday night.

(N.B.—If necessary the Doctor or Nurse will prescribe a different method; but you must in no case omit the doses without a written permission from the Doctor, or, in his absence, from the Senior Nurse.)

2. Between the hours of 9 a.m. and 4.30 p.m. a sun-hat or sun-helmet must be worn when out of doors. After 4.30 p.m. until sunset, and before 9 a.m., a Terai hat should be worn.

3. After sunset members must not sit anywhere unprotected by mosquito netting, unless they happen to be in a house that is not provided with such protection.

Any wilful carelessness in these matters will be reported by the Senior Nurse of the Station to the Bishop, and by the Bishop to the Medical Board in London, and will be counted against the Member when up for examination before returning to Africa.

Approved by the Bishop, July, 1908.

In 1924, 3,461 cases were recorded as treated, 76 were Europeans but only one died. Packets of quinine sulphate (three five grain doses) were on sale in Post Offices for one penny, and 1,343 packets were sold."Sanitary gangs were employed to clear standing water in the township although the results were unsatisfactory."

In 1932 three blood transfusions were given to Europeans with blackwater fever, and other residents were grouped (using the old 1-4 system) so that they could be called upon as volunteers. A synthetic antimalarial, Atebrin, was used with encouraging results.

In 1940, 19·5% of European in-patients (74 cases) were admitted for malaria, but only 8·4% of Africans (1,299 cases).The treatment of blackwater fever had improved with intravenous fluids being given, although the hot colonic irrigations also used sound odd to us today.

The discovery of potent insecticides in the 1940s, together with the introduction of better synthetic antimalarials, seemed to open the way for the possible eradication of the disease, at least in some areas of the world. Alas, the development of insecticide resistance by mosquitoes and antimalarial resistant organisms put an end to this rosy picture in the 1960s.

An estimate of the incidence per 1,000 in 1955, the Malaria Rate was: Africans:2, Asians:6, Europeans:19.5. In 1973 a WHO survey showed that 35% of the people with positive smears had no symptoms at the time. It was suggested that pregnant mothers and infants under five years should take prophylactic chloroquine (discovered in 1960), and also spraying with DDT (that remained active for sometime) should be carried out.

Relentlessly the disease continues to be a major cause of death in children (around 10% of deaths), and a major cause of admission to hospital in adults. Its contribution to ill health, anaemia, and feeling 'half dead', is less easy to measure but it must be considerable. Ten years ago, resistance to chloroquine, the most available anti-malarial, was thought to be a theoretical rather than a practical problem; but within five years resistant strains were emerging. In some areas over 50% of cases of malaria do not respond fully to this drug. Luckily, widespread resistance to quinine does not yet seem to have developed, although it has been used for so long. Today it is usually effective for the sick patient not responding to the more modern and expensive drugs.

The long term hope for the eradication of the disease probably lies in the development of effective vaccines. This is much more difficult in the case of Malaria, Bilharzia, and Sleeping Sickness, than in diseases caused by a simple bacteria or virus. The malarial parasites are able to change their outer coats to which the antibodies must stick to be effective. The hope for a breakthrough lies in the distant future.

Livingstone showed respect to African doctors and suggested their opinions may be relevant. Today, many patients coming to the hospitals bear the scarification marks on their bodies, showing the Sing'anga has been there first.

The Sing'anga, or traditional herbalist, is obvious in local markets and outside hospitals, with his collection of roots, leaves, concoctions and animal parts. They are easily accessible; a writer estimated there was one herbalist per 300 persons in the Domasi area. The increasing pressure of population is causing some medicinal herbs, like some indigenous trees, to become scarce.

They will be consulted for a broad spectrum of troubles from 'mimba'(tummy ache), to cures for infertility, and charms for warding off illness. He will charge, often in kind, and some sing'angas may have wards for inpatient treatment. There is today a registered Society of Traditional Herbalists.

There is no doubt that some mankhwala (African medicine) from plants have pharmacological actions, producing purging, vomiting, and uterine contractions. Control of dosage is a problem, and serious, even fatal results are encountered. One plant,the Kombe arrow and fish poison, in small doses has a stimulating action, like digitalis, on the heart. It was exported to Britain by Mr. Buchanan in the 1890s.

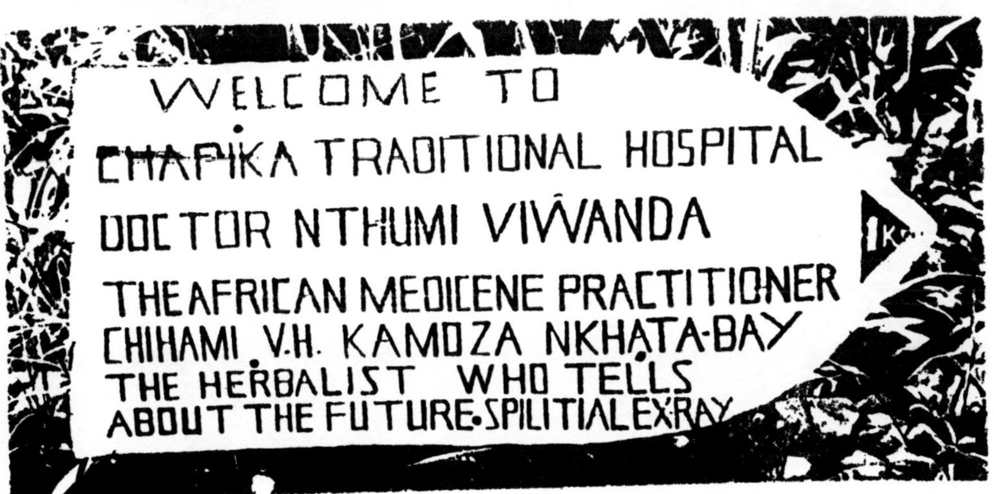

Illus. See also p.127

Dr.Kerr Cross at Karonga (1894) commented favourably on the traditional treatment of fractures by splinting. Leaves and charcoal paste were used to dress wounds and ulcers, probably with beneficial effects. Dr.Elmslie confessed he was astonished on a number of occasions at the results of local medicines.

Less valuable, but also used in Europe, was the dry cupping using the horn of an antelope. This was applied to the skin, a straw was inserted through a hole, the air sucked out, and the hole sealed with beeswax. This produced a weal of blood beneath the skin. Blood letting was used (as it was in Europe) with probable detrimental effects. Rubbing plants and ash into scarifications is very common even today. It is surprising how infrequently these wounds become infected. Steaming of the body and inducing sweating in a hut with a fire, had their parallels in European medicine. There is strong faith in the value of injections, there is even a proprietary pill called 'Jection Pill'.

2   DAILY TIMES TUESDAY MAY 8, 1990

Malawi

Do not bewitch your patients, advises herbalists

TRADITIONAL healers in the country have been urged to encourage their patients to observe rules of hygiene. The call was made on Friday by the national executive chairman of the Traditional Healers Association in Malawi, Mr. █████████.

Mr. █████████ made the call when he addressed traditional healers at Mwanza *Boma* at a meeting which he also spoke against the practice, by the herbalist, of bewitching their patients who failed to pay for services rendered.

"Do not bewitch your patients. You are there to heal and not to kill," he advised.

He said the government had allowed traditional healers to practise alongside trained medical practitioners as part of an attempt to achieve a healthy nation.

The chairman also warned the healers against false claims that they know how to cure Aids. He said the Aids virus had no known cure and that the best the traditional healers could do was to help the government mobilise the people against immoral habits.

█████████ advised the herbalists to practice under the authority of the government and not without licence.

Speaking at the same meeting, the Mwanza district Party chairman, Mr. █████████, called for honesty among traditional healers in appreciation of what the government had done to legalise their practices. —Mana

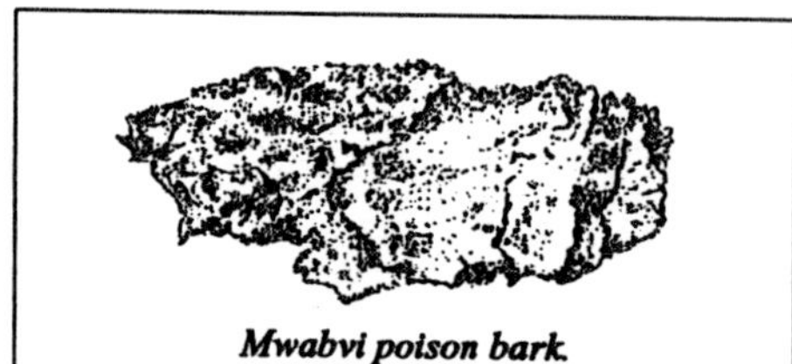

Mwabvi poison bark.

Today, the fear of witchcraft and of being bewitched is very real, but it was more in evidence in days gone by. The Nchimi is a diviner/witch doctor who specializes in this field. To become a nchimi, one has to be possessed. He is able to bewitch or remove spells.

To some extent the nchimi has replaced the old mwabvi (muave) trial by ordeal. Mwabvi is a poison from the tree Erythrophloem guiniense and was given to suspects to drink. If they vomited and survived, they were considered innocent; if they died their guilt was proven. "The number killed by the muave cup cannot be estimated" wrote Dr.Elmslie amongst the Ngoni. At times, the poison was given to animals in a suspect's place.

Johnston recalled how he, Colonel Edwards, and Sharpe, had to wait anxiously for the Mbwavi ordeal result on a chicken or goat, as a suspicious tribe tested the good faith of the strangers. How delighted they were to see the "fowl eject the noxious dose from its crop or the goat refuse the bolus". The Mwabvi ordeal was made illegal in 1911.

Dr.Elmslie gave some accurate descriptions of Ngoni witchcraft. The 'Itshanusi' lived upon the fear and credulity of the people. "When it is decided that a person who is sick has been bewitched, the effect on the person is very marked, he becomes resigned to death and awaits the end." "On many occasions men and women have sought refuge at the Mission Station when accused of witchcraft, and under sentence of death. On one occasion, during a trial which took place at a village near the station, when the Itshanusi was performing his incantations, and condemned a man, he broke away from the crowd and ran towards this house. He was followed by a crowd of men and boys clamouring for his life, and, being overtaken, was clubbed to death before our eyes. His body was ignominiously dragged back to the scene of the trial where it was subjected to gross indignities."

"In nearly every hut a bundle of poison bark would be found hid away in the roof against the need to use it. Family and other quarrels were finally adjusted by resort to the ordeal. Numberless cases were treated at the Dispensary when more sober reflections made them seek an emetic (sulphate of zinc and water)." "Three months previously Chief Chikusi had sent his Sing'anga with the muave to test a village's subjection. Everybody had drunk it, including children above 10 years old. Seven died but no children."

"Only today a man came rushing into the mission yard appealing to Dr.Elmslie for help, as he had taken a long and strong pull from the poison gourd. One of his wives and himself having had a disagreement, it was mutually decided that they both take the test. The wife infused the poisonous decoction of bark and took the first drink, and immediately commenced to vomit, a sure indication that she was in the right. But the husband was not so fortunate, for having finished the potion, it did not react as he had hoped, and fearing death, repented of what he had done, and made for the Mission House, where a prompt emetic put him out of danger." (James Johnston at Bandawe 1892)

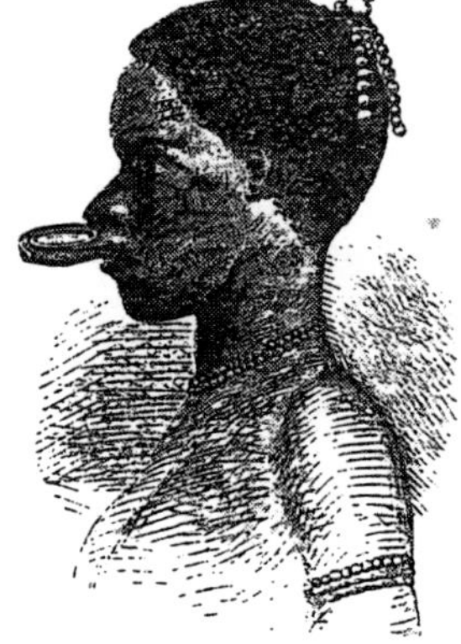

Pelele

Tattooing for beautification is dying out in Malaŵi, and is only seen in the older people; the pelele, a lip plug inserted in a slit in the upper lip, vanished at the beginning of this century.

There are many taboos and beliefs related to childbirth, pregnancy, and menstruation. An obstructed labour may denote adultery, and eggs are not eaten during pregnancy in some parts of the country. For many village women even now it is the traditional midwife or 'Myamba' who will advise and deliver them. Some have had extra training in hospitals, and have knowledge of hygiene and when to refer patients or babies to hospital. They are respected and often wealthy members of the community, and may have small waiting wards.

Most rural babies will have a string tied around the waist with a charm on it, some leaves sewn into a small pouch. Powder is put into small animal horns as a charm to ward off evil or bring good luck in various aspects of life.

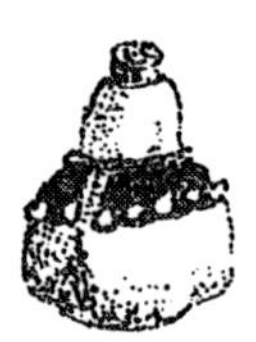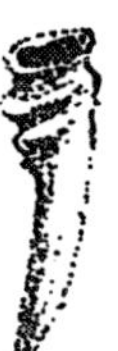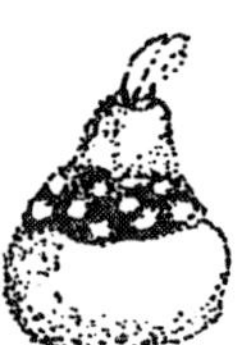

Nsupa (Gourds) and a Nyanga (horn) containing various ingredients to bewitch or prevent bewitching. Blantyre Museum

Chief Msamara was imprisoned in Fort Johnston in the 1890s. Friends brought him a horn of medicine to make him invisible. He took all his clothes off (they could not be rendered invisible), and attempted to walk out of the prison. The Sikh sentries at bayonet point forced him to retire to his cell where he explained he must have been walking in his sleep. The next night he was found dead, with the empty horn in his hand and all his clothes removed.

The recent Aids epidemic has given rise to an increase in herbal medicine and witchcraft throughout Africa, as scientific medicine can so far offer no help.

5   DR. and MRS. ROBERT LAWS (served 1875-1928)

"The love of Christ constraineth us."

Robert Laws.

"When God wills something to be done, He will give us the means to do it"
(Robert Laws)

In 1874, the Church of Scotland released the Rev. Dr.Robert Laws to go to Lake Nyasa for two years only. He stayed for 53 years to achieve some of the most impressive medical mission work in Africa.

He was a carpenter's son and he attended Miss Melville's Sunday School at St. Nicholas Church, Aberdeen. Five other famous missionaries were in this class, including his future wife, Margaret Gray.

At 12 he started work as an apprentice carpenter, and at 15 committed his life to be a missionary:"if I am to be of greatest use, I must be fully qualified in every way". He entered Aberdeen University to study arts, theology, and medicine, and won the Botany prize. In 1870 he nearly died of smallpox. He qualified as a doctor in 1874, and at once joined the pioneer Livingstonia Mission party, led by Captain E.D. Young R.N. and embarked for Africa. On board was the *Ilala*, a specially designed boat in sections that could be carried around the Shire River Cataracts, and assembled again on the upper reaches of the river.

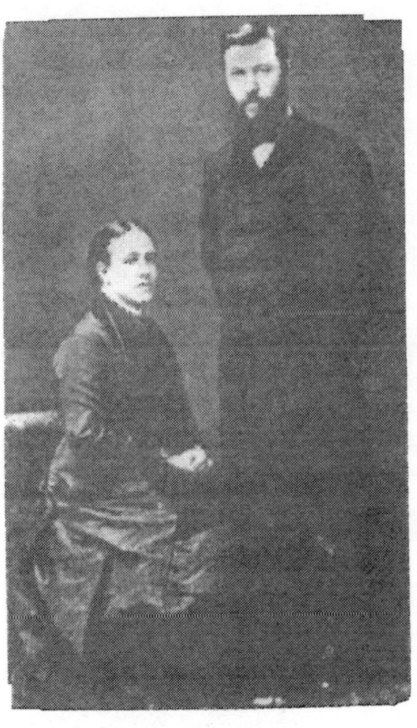

Dr and Mrs R Laws

CAPE MACLEAR 1875-81

With six other artisan Scots, they sailed into Lake Nyasa on the steamer *Ilala* on October 12th 1875, and landed at Cape Maclear. Laws wrote home: "Livingstonia is begun, though at present it is only a piece of canvas stretched between two trees."

Immediately they set to, to build a bungalow 50 feet by 25 feet. On the first day 200 trees were cut down. Laws worked with the rest, digging holes, felling trees, sawing, thatching, claying, planting vegetables, washing clothes, and tending the sick. By November 9th, as the first thunderstorms broke, this house was ready.

Laws then set off with Young to make the first complete circumnavigation of Lake Nyasa. They found it was 350 miles long, and "on the shores of Lake Nyasa we have villages and towns with inhabitants of 200 to 10,000." At Bandawe they were met by the five Chiefs who had greeted Dr.Livingstone.

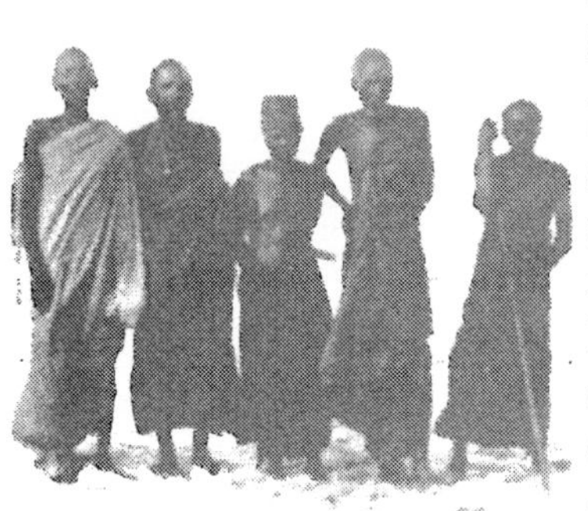

The Five Chiefs at Bandawe

Back at Cape Maclear in December 1875, malaria was rife, and Dr.Laws suffered 15 attacks in a few months. Often he had to crawl from his mattress to tend others. The roof leaked. Leopards and lions roared around at night, crocodiles and hippos prowled the beach, and elephants trampled their gardens.

The slave trade was their worst problem. About 30,000 slaves were then being transported across Lake Nyasa each year. Dr.Laws perceived its commercial cause; Africans lacked other exportable commodities. "Our Chiefs sold us to buy cotton and guns from the Arabs".

Cape Maclear was surrounded by such chiefs. Chief Jumbe had made Nkhota Kota with 5,000 people into the biggest slave depot in Central Africa; Chief Mponda at Mangochi was continually capturing slaves and selling them; and on the other side of the Lake, Chief Makanjira was building more dhows to transport them. In 1876, Arab slavers came and seized some Mission workers at Cape Maclear.

Dr.Laws wrote home: "My work is not to put down the slave trade, but I never felt my blood boil as it did today...I wish I could shoulder my rifle and defend these poor creatures. Mr.Young felt like a caged lion, for the thousandth time he wished he had Government powers to put an end to this horrid traffic in human flesh and blood."

Five months after arriving, Dr.Laws did the first surgical operation with chloroform at Cape Maclear. It established a permanent trust between him and the Nyasa people.(See chapter on surgery). He looked after each patient with meticulous care, and a few of his own case notes survive from Cape Maclear. There are notes about the disease symptoms of a woman from Chimlolo's village, about fever affecting the schoolboys, and about an operation for Zumani's tumour.

In September 1877, Dr.Black arrived to take charge of the Mission, in a party with John Gunn (farmer), Robert Ross (engineer), A.C. Miller (weaver), and Dr.James Stewart. Black survived only 7 months at Cape Maclear before dying of malaria. Then Shadrach Nguna and John Mackay (boatman) died of tuberculosis and Laws tended them devotedly.

Robert Laws then bravely summoned his childhood sweetheart, Margaret Gray, from Aberdeen, and they were married in the little thatched church at Blantyre on August 28th 1878. She was the first European lady to live by the Lake. At Cape Maclear the Africans welcomed her by dancing for two nights, and she transformed the rough Mission room with a tablecloth, flowers, and a cosy lamp. She was a born teacher and at once started classes for the girls. Dr.Laws soon needed her help in giving chloroform.

Mrs.Laws' trust in her husband's skill equalled everyone else's. In December 1879, they sailed together to explore the north end of Lake Nyasa, naming Amelia Bay after her sister, and taking a small elephant on board. She slept on deck and in heavy rain spread her skirt over the engine. One dark stormy night, the Doctor went forward to where she stood clinging to the rigging: "Well, are you afraid?" "No...because you are at the helm."

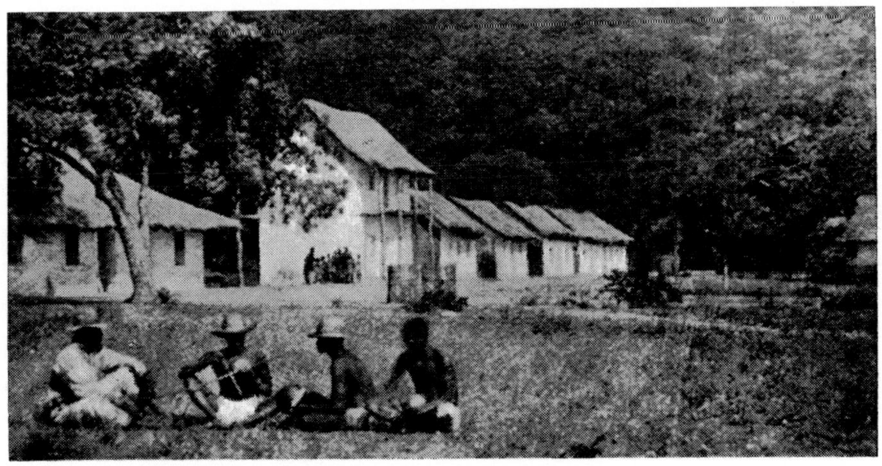

Double-decker and Cape Maclear mission.

Returning to Cape Maclear in 1880, they were both very ill with malaria, and then, the Master of the *Ilala,* Captain Benzie, and John Gunn from Caithness both suddenly died of fever. The Doctor tended Gunn for three days: " the temperature rapidly increased, he vomited blood (coffee grounds), petechial spots appeared rapidly over his body. About 1p.m. he began talking in Gaelic, and spoke no more English, nor was he conscious afterwards. At 5.5 p.m. he passed away. Sometime afterwards the thermometer in his axilla registered 109·9° Fahrenheit."

The Laws were devastated by these deaths. There were now five Mission graves at Cape Maclear. Yet Dr.Laws could see a distinct way forward. In 1880 he treated 776 patients in his dispensary (495 new ones). The school started by Dr.Black with 17 children had grown to 90 scholars by 1881.

Robert Laws perceived that both primary school education and Christian marriage would be the foundation of real progress. He conducted several marriages at Cape Maclear for couples with genuinely monogamous intentions.

"The Christian home, begun by the marriage of a man and a woman, suited to each other, is the nursery of the Church, and its purity must be held inviolate".

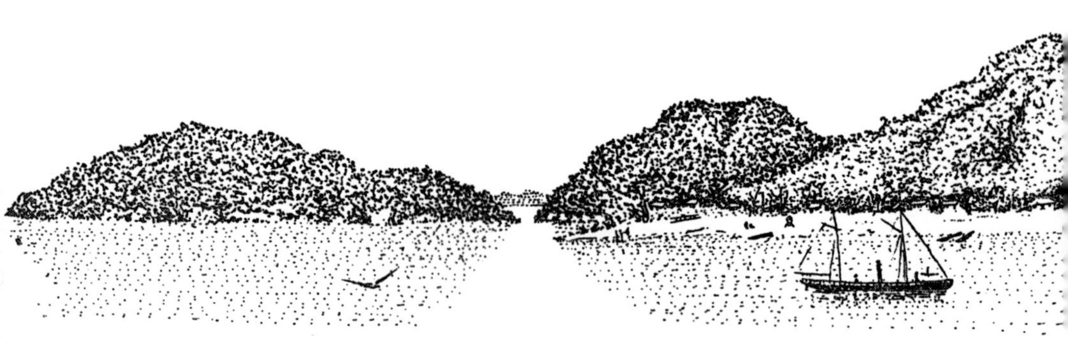

Panorama of Cape Maclear (after Elton) showing the Ilala

BANDAWE 1881-94

On March 29th 1881 Dr.and Mrs.Laws sailed north from Cape Maclear to go to the Tonga, Tumbuka, and Ngoni, people who wanted their help.

Captain E.D. Young R.N. had first encountered the Ngoni by the Shire River in 1877. They were a branch of the Zulu tribe which had migrated to escape from Chaka's butchery, and still spoke the Zulu language. Young described them as "a merciless horde, they have been trained to fight at close quarter with the assegai and spear; with Zulu discipline they advanced in true military style, all 300 of them...I was listened to with deepest attention... they were much pleased and trusted that we would not confine ourselves to these southern tribes, but would come north to them. They desired one of the British to visit their great Chief who lived far north."

In 1879, the Chief M'mbelwa had summoned Dr.Laws to his cattle kraal at Njuyu, four days walking from Nkhata Bay. This first encounter between the Ngoni people and Europeans was later recalled: "we Ngoni children were hidden away because it was feared the white men would hurt us...the people believed Lobarti (Robert) was a fish because he lived in the Lake on a steamer."

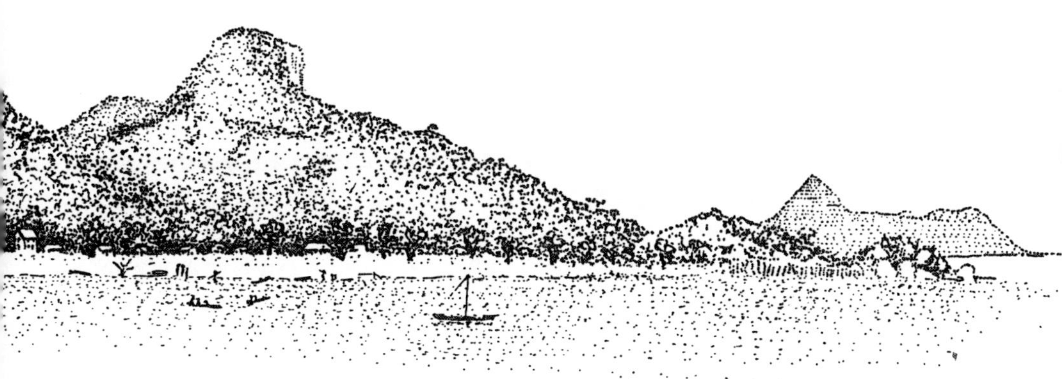

The Mission including doubledecker house, the Herga and Otter Point.

The next day Chief M'mbelwa at last appeared to a huge assembly of warriors shouting "Bayete"(hail). He looked slowly at Dr.Laws, and at once a bond of mutual respect was established between these two strong men. This legendary friendship was to be the foundation of progress in Nyasaland. As a Scottish Highlander and clansman, Laws understood these proud Ngoni hill people.

"We are disappointed that you have not come and settled with us Ngoni. Why do you like the Lake? Can you milk fish?" Laws promised to send Mission teachers to them in due course. Before he left Njuyu Village, a lion was killed and the warriors danced the fearsome Lion Dance in celebration.

In October 1881, Dr.and Mrs.Laws, with only two other missionaries, settled by the Lake at Bandawe, and hurried to build the first wattle and daub house and plant vegetables before the rains. Four Tonga Chiefs, Marengo, Chikoko, Chimbano, and Kampala, had welcomed their settlement. Within half an hour, the school attracted 40 children, and dozens of patients came seeking help from Dr.Laws. A red cross flag was hoisted to show when his clinic was open.

In 1882 he had 3,104 patients of whom 2,304 were treated at Bandawe. Most of these were surgical emergencies, for the cruelty of nature and of man kept him busy. One man who had been seized by a crocodile, had deep wounds stuffed with charcoal and burned leaves; another had his filled with sand, this being a traditional form of treatment.

A man whose thigh had been broken by a bullet and needed an amputation asked: "how shall I hoe my garden with only one leg?" "better hoe your garden with one leg than go to your grave with two" replied the Doctor grimly. Most of this work was done in simple conditions, often out of doors.

Dr.Laws described a case at Bandawe in 1882: "One of the greatest surprises to the Africans was the use of chloroform... lest superstitious ideas might be circulated about what was done, I asked two Chiefs to be present at the operation. The amputation of the hand was simple enough, but the tumour on the face required very delicate dissection under prolonged anaesthesia. During the operation I glanced over my shoulder at the two Chiefs, tall strong men they were, holding their hands over their mouths in amazement at the woman sleeping quietly while I was occupied."

Suddenly Bandawe Mission was besieged by 500 fugitives from the marauding Ngoni who were threatening to attack the Tonga. In April 1882 Dr.Laws, with Dr.Hannington and William Koyi (the Zulu missionary), went again to visit Chief M'mbelwa at Njuyu. Laws asked to meet all the sub-chiefs and waited nine days for all these Indunas to arrive.

They were addressed first by the handsome Chief Mtwalo who asked Dr.Laws to leave the Lake and settle in the hills with the Ngoni. Laws, very ill with fever, said he wished to preach Christianity so that all the people might be happy and strong. The Mission wanted to teach children how to read the Bible and to give medicines to the sick. This would be better than war. Chief Mtwalo was impressed and Chief M'mbelwa made a formal pledge of protection for the Tonga of Bandawe ratified by an exchange of cattle and blankets.

Then Dr.Hannington collapsed with cerebral malaria, and an urgent message was sent to Bandawe. Mrs.Laws brought Mrs.Hannington on a rough and dangerous five day journey, going over the Viphya Mountains, to Njuyu. They passed wild animals and Mrs.Laws' neck was severely sunburnt and never fully recovered.

Dr.Laws set to, and built a mud hut for the Hanningtons in Njuyu Village. He and Mrs.Laws slept in a tent beside it for several weeks, as the patient hovered between life and death. During this sojourn, William Koyi began his remarkable work and the hut became the first mission building in Ngoniland.

Back at Bandawe, they were shocked to hear that a missionary party under Dr.Stewart had been attacked whilst landing at Karonga, with many Cape Maclear Christians killed.

In December 1883, utterly exhausted, Dr.and Mrs.Laws departed from Bandawe for their first home leave in Scotland.

Laws made a formal report to the Church of Scotland: "The increasing confidence of the Africans in the medical missionary is shown by the fact that in 1882 there were 3,300 attendances at Bandawe, and in 1883 about 7,000, while in 1884 they exceeded 10,000. The marauding Ngoni can respect and trust as a friend the medical missionary, so a doctor has been appointed to each of the Ngoni districts." Dr. Elmslie and Dr. Kerr Cross were despatched to the Livingstonia Mission.

In June 1886, the Laws embarked for Africa again, accompanied by the prospective brides of these doctors. In August, steaming precariously up the Shire River in the re-floated *Lady Nyasa*, Mrs.Laws lay on a stretcher on the forward deck. The boat stopped at midnight in the steaming malarial Elephant

Marsh, surrounded by wild animals. The Doctor was beside her with candles casting a dim light around. Presently she gave birth to a daughter, Amelia Nyasa Laws.

Back at Bandawe, malaria was endemic. Amy,"a pale faced wee body" was at the point of death. Mrs.Laws was severely ill, Dr. and Mrs.Elmslie were both prostrated at Njuyu, and at Mwiniwanda newly married Mrs.Kerr Cross died. Dr. Laws rose weakly from his sick bed to tend Mr.Swinney, the pioneer missionary from Likoma Island, who also died.

Then news came that famine was causing the Ngoni to prepare to attack the Tonga. Dr. Laws packed his medical equipment and prepared to sail away with his family. But the Tonga Chiefs came to insist that the Laws must stay at Bandawe, and took away their boats. In the quiet night the Doctor saw the shadowy sentries placed around his house, whilst Mrs.Laws, cradling Amy in the kitchen, sang softly "the Lord is my Shepherd, I shall not want."

Soon Chief M'mbelwa summoned Dr. Laws to another great Indaba in his Njuyu cattle kraal. With the promise of a Scottish doctor for Chief Mtwalo's Village (Ekwendeni), peace was agreed. As Dr. Laws departed, huge Ngoni regiments came marching in from the north.

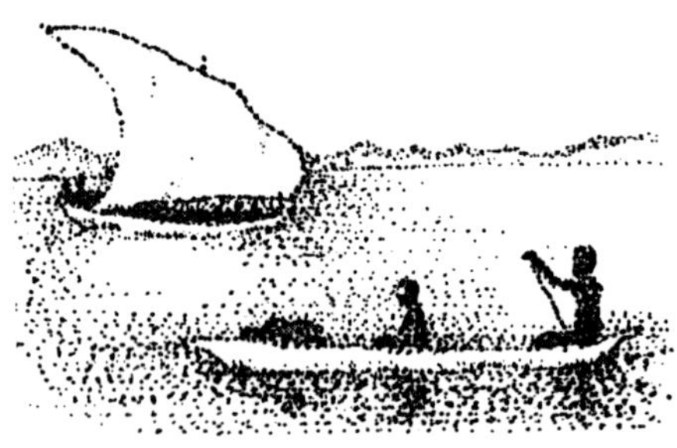

Dhow and Dugout

The slave trade was still in full swing. The missionaries were constantly seeing dhows crossing the Lake from Deep Bay(Chilumba) packed with victims, many of them starving boys and girls. In 1887 the Arab slavers, led by their Chief, Mlozi, began a series of atrocities against the Nkonde people, culminating in the terrible massacre at Kambwe Lagoon. British forces led by Captain Lugard attacked these Arabs, and Dr. Laws tended some of the casualties.

In 1887 Captain Lugard wrote: "late in the evening we arrived at Bandawe and I met Dr. and Mrs.Laws and shared their generous hospitality. Dr. Laws is a remarkable man, and his well worn library, including literature on a wide range of subjects evidenced the extent of his reading. To his careful observation is due much of the knowledge we have both of the Lake and the mainland."

Tonga and Tumbuka memories of Robert Laws at Bandawe were: "Dotolozi (Dr. Laws) came when there was great trouble...we were afraid of being sold as slaves, every headman sold people to get cloth and ammunition. The

Ngoni had control of the district and we had to pay a tax of food ...wars...fights".

"Dotolozi was a charmer; he charmed the whole district so that the Ngoni would not come near us."

"The Doctor was a tall man with black hair. We called him Sing'anga wankura, the great doctor. When he came, he stopped all fighting between the Chiefs."

In 1890 the Consul Harry Johnston visited Bandawe and wrote: "Dr. Laws is a doctor of medicine and a practised surgeon with a well stocked dispensary. In order to teach others, he has become a practised engineer, carpenter, joiner, printer, farrier, boat builder, and druggist."

LIVINGSTONIA at KONDOWE 1894-1928

In 1894, the Laws, with Yuriah Chirwa, at last moved their work to a hill station at Kondowe, 4,500 feet above sea level, looking down on Lake Nyasa. The Ngoni people came to help the Mission, levelling roads, building houses, and bringing their children to school. The Laws' first house was blown down by a tornado the night after its completion.

Rinderpest swept the district in 1895, killing the cattle, so hungry animals started attacking humans. A leopard leapt through a glass window of their house as Mrs.Laws was sitting in the room.

Livingstonia Crest

In 1897 the Doctor treated 9,917 patients of whom 7,392 were surgical. Many had been mauled by wild animals, especially lions which would jump through the grass roof of a hut at night.

"One case...a leopard attacked some men in a garden while they were working, and four of them were badly mauled. The teacher at the village advised they should be taken at once to Livingstonia Hospital, but the Chief forbade it. Next day he allowed the transference of three, so their friends made hammocks of nets tied to poles and carried them three days journey to the Hospital. Their wounds had not been dressed, and when they arrived, I was conscious of the odour 50 yards away; while so much sand and charcoal made from burnt leaves had been put on the wounds that it took 3 hours hard work to clean them. To our surprise, they all recovered well." (Robert Laws)

Then the "Jiggers" epidemic arrived, causing bad ulcers. One day Laws removed 12 of the fleas from his own toes.

Visitors to Livingstonia in 1900 wrote "We missed our boat": "Here's Dr. Laws. And surely he was there, tired after his descent, all kindness and sympathy. Soon we were all drinking longed for cups of tea. Mrs.Laws in her accustomed thoughtful way, had sent a plentiful store of good things down. Soon we commenced the climb, there was no road in those days, the Doctor making us use the machila. It was terrible, at times so steep you felt you must topple over backwards.

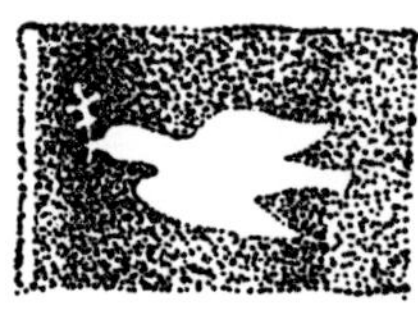

Livinstonia Flag

As we repeatedly stopped to regain our breath, Dr. Laws would come up, and tell us of the old days, pointing out in the far distance below spot after spot made historic by Rhodes, Stewart, and many others.

When we reached their house, after 4 or 5 hours climb, Mrs.Laws was there to greet us. There was something specially prepared for baby Margaret, and hot soup for ourselves.

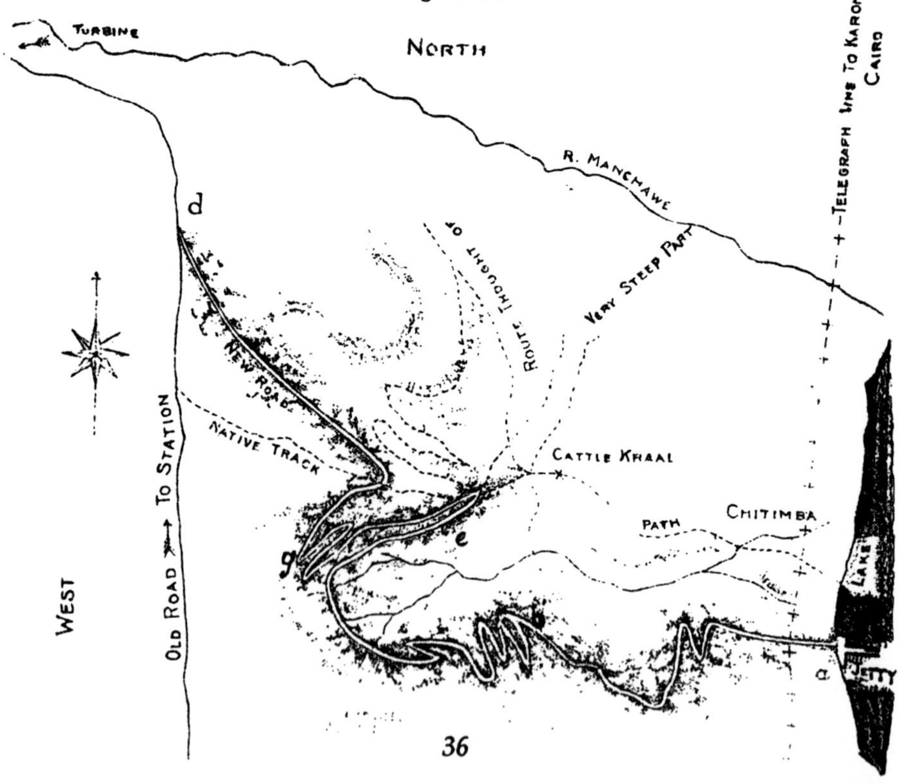

That evening the whole staff gathered together, and we sang hymns to our hearts' content, Dr. and Mrs.Laws enjoying as much as anyone. Some said 'It was a good thing you missed the steamer.' Dr. Laws never seems to be in a hurry. No man sees to his work more conscientiously, every letter is answered quickly, thoroughly, and with unfailing courtesy. He stays up to the early hours of the morning to finish his correspondence."

As the century turned, Laws brought new technology to Khondowe. In 1899 he attended a course on electricity and engineering at Heriot Watt College, Edinburgh, and then returned to construct a piped water supply from the Manchewe River, and a hydro-electric dynamo from the Manchewe Falls. The first electric light in Nyasaland was switched on at his Mission in 1905. He also constructed the famous Longmuir Road from Khondowe down to the Lakeshore, which descends 2,300 feet in 3 miles. It is still a good road today. He built his own traditional Scottish Stone House at this Mission, and organized the African Transcontinental Telegraph Line to encompass Livingstonia.

The essential wisdom of Dr. Laws' policy lay in his approach to ignorance, poverty, and disease. He could see that human progress depended on the problem of ignorance being tackled first. Primary schooling for children had first priority in all his work.

Livingstonia Education					
Year	Schools	Scholars	Year	Schools	Scholars
1881	2	147	1898	108	10,838
1885	6	558	1900	123	16,000
1889	21	2,422	1905	200	22,000
1893	40	3,230	1908	500	30,000
1895	51	4,501	1925	917	53,000
1896	71	7,641			

In 1905 the Church of Scotland could not understand why the total cost of running 200 schools was only £1,300 per year. Laws himself went into the villages to build these simple mud and wattle schools, and the only equipment needed was a few alphabet boards and a slate and chalk for each child. The local teachers were trained at Livingstonia. The door to better health and prosperity was opened to thousands by these mission schools, and many of the Livingstonia pupils proceeded to distinguished careers.

Dr. Laws also planned medical services for North Nyasaland with well equipped hospitals from which staff could tour the surrounding district. In two years 1903-5, thirteen Livingstonia hospitals were built as local "self-help" projects; together with sixteen more dispensaries, and 83,043 patients were treated.

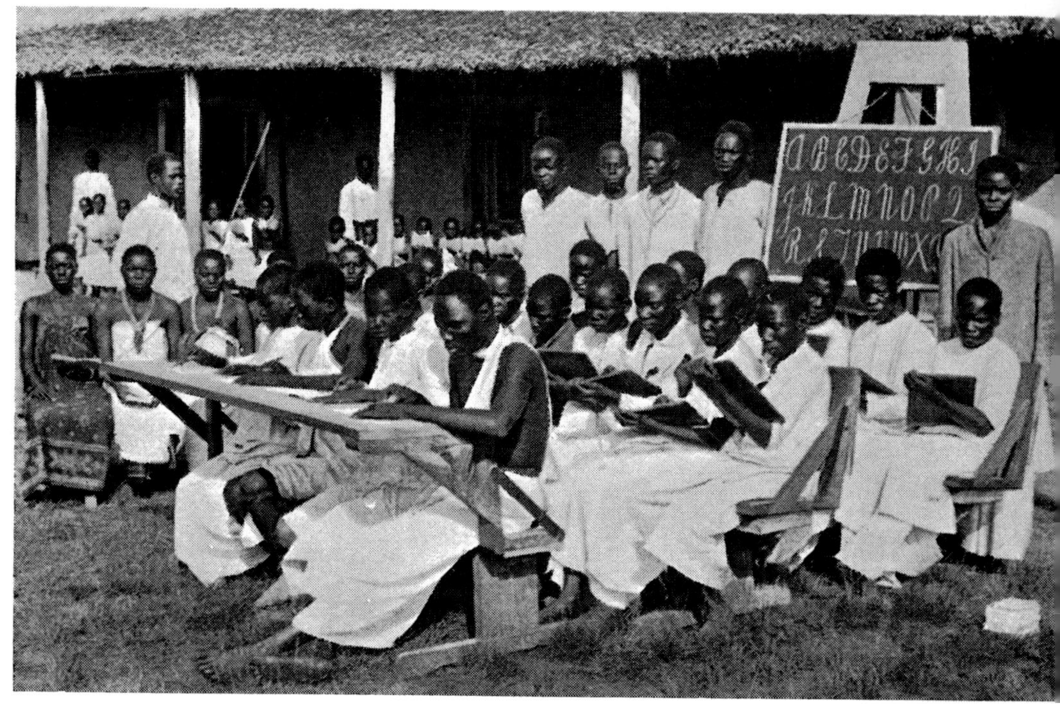

Bandawe Mission Senior Class 1900.

One case in 1909 was not so lucky. The Livingstonia News reported "a small snake attended at the consultation room the other evening , with a fatal result to itself."

In 1905 Robert Laws went on a missionary ulendo to south Tanganyika with Dr. Chisholm, who wrote: "any friends at home who had anxiety about his undertaking a journey of 1,500 miles would have had their minds set at rest if they had seen him march up to 20 miles a day, sleep one night in the open with no ill effects, and be carried in his machila less often than those who have been in the country 3 years instead of 30."

He was also busy at home. Often a knock would come on the door as he was thinking of retiring, and he would spend hours in a distant hut, sitting beside a smoking fire as he cared for a sick person. He would openly denounce the witch doctors in a village.

In 1904 the Ngoni gathered in their thousands, Chiefs, Indunas, and Impis of warriors, with shields and spears, to see the British Governor Sharpe with Dr. Laws. They had come to surrender their old wild way of life, to submit to authority and taxation. With the Doctor's help, the Ngoni agreed to be a part of the Nyasaland Protectorate, with their own police.

A Nyasa plea reached Scotland in 1908; "if Dr. Laws is to stay in Scotland, the whole of our land will weep, and catch him, and stop his loads going. Dr. and Mrs.Laws have been given to us by God. They are not Europeans now, they are Africans."

Lord Overtoun who died in 1909, had given £50,000 to Livingstonia, and donated £1,000 per year to pay salaries. Rarely has money been better spent. Another grant of £5,000 in memory of David Gordon, was used to build Dr. Laws' first

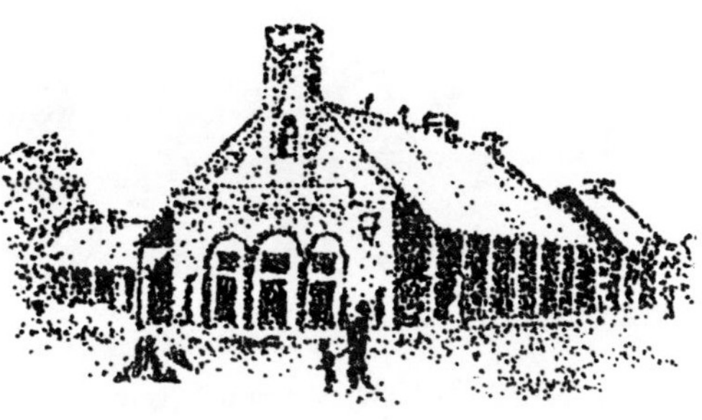

David Gordon Memorial Hospital (D.G.M.).

hospital, designed exactly to suit local needs, in 1911.

"Umudala uze umuthi" (Ngoni proverb) "Old age has no medicine"

The outbreak of the Great War caused Dr. Laws to fear his work might be jeopardized. Berlin missionaries in Tanganyika wrote to ask him to prevent hostilities in East Africa. He did manage to establish some humanitarian measures in a meeting between German and British army commanders.

In September 1914, German soldiers crossed the Songwe River and attacked Karonga. They were repulsed after desperate fighting. Then the Livingstonia Mission was slowly depleted of its staff: doctors were conscripted into the army, teachers were drafted off as scouts, interpreters, and transport leaders. Every boat on Lake Nyasa hurried north, and endless files of soldiers and porters were marching northwards. The Mission had to provide food, oxen, printing, planking, engineering, and other supplies to the war effort. Bandawe Hospital was taken over by the army; many Livingstonia schools closed, training ceased, and a stricken Europe stopped sending aid to Africa.

By 1916, the Mission reported:"more than half our staff are away in war service; four of our wards are at the service of the Nyasaland Field Force." Soldier cases were mostly dysentery and malaria. Later disabled Africans struggled home via Livingstonia from the war zone.

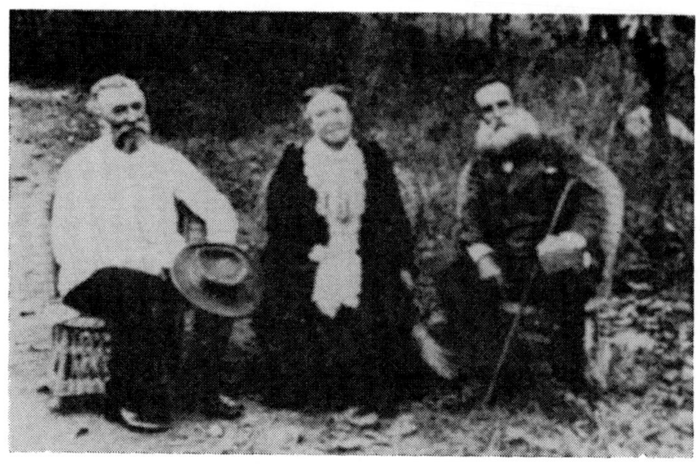

Dr. and Mrs Laws and Rev. J. Moffat 1902.

Dr. and Mrs.Laws were in charge of the Livingstonia mission work alone in 1917. When serious surgical cases arrived, she gave the chloroform again, as she had done 40 years before. They now had to take over the work of the Berlin and Moravian missions abandoned by the Germans as well. Mrs.Laws had a serious illness that year, and never properly recovered.

Robert Laws, always modest and taciturn, gave a rare interview to a reporter in 1920, and spoke with emotion: "Mrs.Laws has been my constant help during all these years. I owe her more than I can tell to her. She has been an unspeakable comfort. We have come through perilous times together. Many a night she and I never knew what the morning would bring.

The changes in Central Africa since I entered it are greater than those which came over Scotland in a thousand years.

It is often said that the highest qualifications are not required for the missionary to Africa. The opposite is the case. It needs also the finest character. It is not one's preaching and work that tells on people, but the example of one's life."

After 42 years of married life in Nyasaland, Margaret Laws was hurried home to Edinburgh in 1921, and died.

Robert Laws, robust in old age, continued his work. He greeted a visitor wearing huge boots: "Do you know what Livingstone looked to first when he began his journey? It was Captain Young who told me: his boots and his mosquito net". At the age of 70, Dr. Laws went on ulendo to the Henga

Valley, walking mile after mile through the long grass with a steady swing. He would sleep rough and carry on through a heavy storm. Not until 1924 did Livingstonia recover from the problems of the War. Progress that might have been made: disease control programmes, training courses for hospital staff and even for doctors, were probably delayed for decades. Financial support was much reduced from an impoverished postwar Europe.

For 50 years Dr. Laws had been training medical assistants, and he now saw this work securely established in Nyasaland. A National Approved Course was approved in 1926, and the National Medical Council was formed to register qualified hospital staff. The first Medical Assistant on this Register was James Msiska from Livingstonia Medical College.

In 1927 Dr. Laws had an operation with a spinal anaesthetic in Edinburgh. Before the surgeon began he said, "I have never operated on anyone without a word of prayer".... so all had to stop while Dr. Laws commended himself and the surgeon and staff to God's care and guidance.

As Robert Laws left Nyasaland in 1928 there were many tributes:

"He has appeared to Africans as a man of daring spirit. He had a message to deliver and that he accomplished. He is a wonderful man in his humility, meekness, patience, and compassion."

"The African attitude to him was remarkable. His presence commanded the situation. "

A Nyasa student commented "He was a very fair man, a very strict disciplinarian, a man of God."

"A word from him was authoritative to all."

Scotsmen noted: "What is most admirable is the quiet, continuous, sustained, work of Dr. Laws."

"In aspect a stalwart Scots farmer, quiet and observant, with the fire of a great passion burning deep in his hazel eyes...a great figure indeed."

Robert Laws died on August 6th 1934 in London. He was buried in the old churchyard of St. Machar, Aberdeen, after a crowded funeral at St. Nicholas' Church.

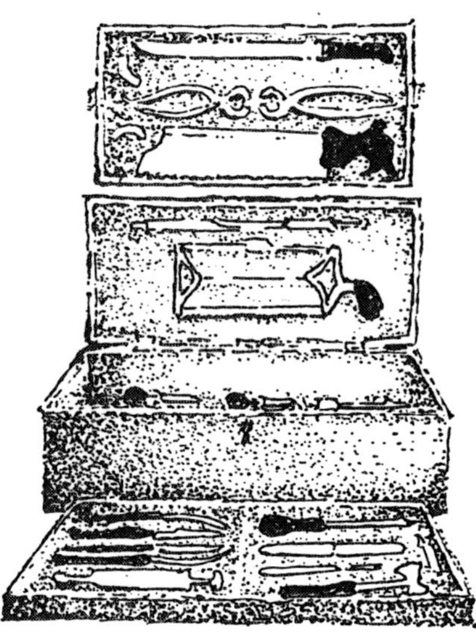

1880 UMCA Surgical Instruments. Lake Malawi Museum, Mangochi

Surgical attention is often the most urgent medical need in the community. The first doctors would all have had a set of pocket surgical instruments. There are many early reports of animal and war wounds and severe infections treated in very primitive conditions.

The first chloroform case in Central Africa was a man named Koomfonjera with a cystic tumour above the left eye. He was first noticed by Dr. Laws at Mponda's Village, an operation was suggested but the patient was afraid. Two days later he was brought by canoe to Cape Maclear and asked for help. On March 2nd 1876, Dr. Laws placed this patient on his dining room table: "Three Africans stood and watched. When the Chloroform was administered (by dripping it on to a cloth held over the patient's mouth and nose), the patient lay still and insensible and the astonishment of the audience knew no bounds: 'Za za, wa wa,' they kept calling. The doctor removed the tumour and by early evening Koomfonjera was doing well. He was soon discharged cured." News spread far and wide and soon many patients appeared.....confidence in surgery was growing, from extracting teeth to serious operations. People called the chloroform 'dying' and would crowd around the building and stand in open mouthed wonder at the surgeon calmly cutting away at a man's body while his African assistants mopped up the blood: "The sooner we get them trained to do this work, the better." (R.Laws).

Karonga 1892 "Also Dr.Poole amputated a number of shattered limbs from the Mpata (slave) war.

"Likoma 1895 "Dr.Howard carried out a successful four hour long operation on a 19 year old boy with mastoiditis (ear infection) threatening to spread to the brain. "Karonga 1907: "A mauled crocodile case, the clavicle and scapular both seen through the wounds in the shoulder. A probe ran along two bare ribs on the right side...13 deep punctured wounds of the right arm from shoulder to palm, into which a foot or two of inch wide gauze could be placed."(Dr. Innes) There were also constant streams of patients with ulcers for dressings.

"Chloroform has been administered at least a dozen times in the year by Pondomani who has been the chloroformist for the past 7 years. One elephantiasis scrotii weighed 53 lbs."(North End 1895 Dr.Kerr Cross).

"Chloroforming never cost me an anxious thought.We have had no accident under chloroform which has been administered in 40 cases during the year."(Bandawe 1897 Dr.Prentice)

Cataract operations (removing an opaque lens under a local cocaine anaesthetic) were among the most dramatic. A degree of sight could be restored to a previously blind man enabling him to find his way along local paths. In 1913, Dr.Prentice carried out four in one week in Kasungu.

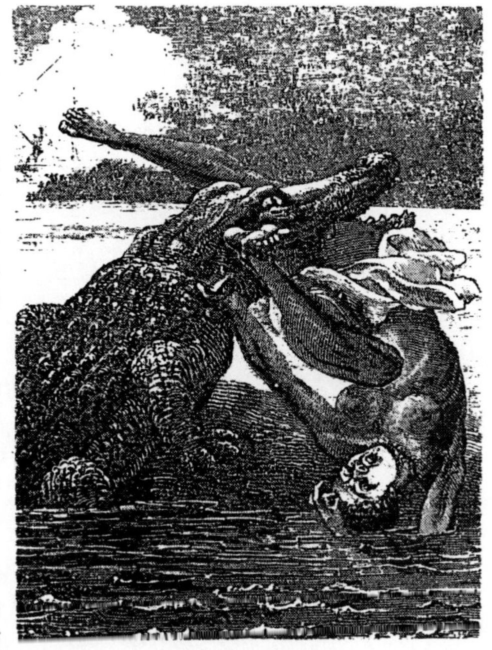

Crocodile attack.

Equipment had to be improvised on occasions: Mulanje Scottish Presbyterian Mission reported in 1894 that there was a raid from Portuguese East Africa on Chisambuka's Village and many gunshot dead and wounded:"We thank H.M.Commissioner for a grant of £25 towards replacing surgical instruments carried off in the raid." However, before the instruments arrived, a Yao with a gangrenous arm came in: "As our surgical instruments have not yet been replaced, the amputating instrument was a pocket knife from Mr. Simpson; for dividing the bone we had a joiner's keyhole saw kindly lent by Mr.Moir...the bone was cut through a little below the shoulder, and the stump is now healing nicely and he has quite given up the idea of dying."

In the north, before the David Gordon Memorial Hospital was opened in 1910 at Livingstonia (Khondowe), reed huts were used as operating theatres. The roof of the D.G.M.Hospital was erected the day before the rains broke that year (three inches in two hours the next day). 93 operations, including such major cases as obstructed hernia and a perforated gastric ulcer, were carried out in 1911.

In 1904, Blantyre Mission had an "up to date operating table, glass top lotions table to which a glass needle box and ligature (suture) trough has just been added, and a handy instrument sterilizer.'

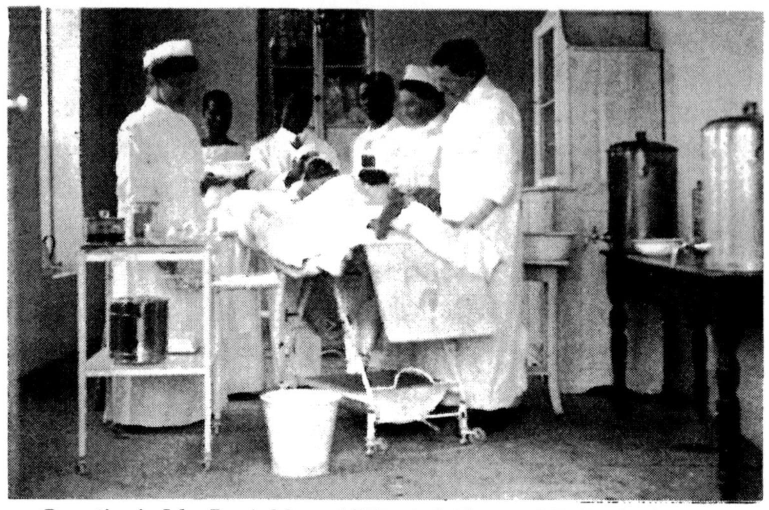

Operation in John Bowie Memorial Hospital, Blantyre Mission (early 1900's)

The belt drives of cotton gins caused some of the first industrial injuries. In 1908 a quarryman at Livingstonia hammered a dynamite cartridge with a stone resulting in the loss of fingertips!

In 1916, Dr.Prentice operated on Jessie at Kasungu: "When Jessie first came to the Mission she was a walking skeleton, only an operation could save her life. In due time Dr.Turner arrived from Bandawe, and after careful consideration and preparations, we tackled the removal of what we knew to be a large abdominal tumour, and we soon found to be a multilocular cyst and purulent at that (probably from the ovary). Jessie's mother sat beside the little path that leads from the operation room to the ward...to the poor old woman her daughter seemed dead.'The maid is not dead but sleepeth' we said as we removed the covering blanket. Jessie's wounds healed by first intention and she left the hospital completely cured."

In 1924 the D.G.M.Hospital carried out 117 major operations and over a thousand minor ones. "The increase in surgical work made big demands on our staff. During the months the hospital was without a nurse, the medical assistants rose gloriously to the occasion and worked well." Two years later "a splendid operating table has arrived and a tremendous boon it has proved."

The early doctors were jacks of all trades and would turn their hands to anything although there is a striking lack of reports of obstetric cases. In 1927, the first X-ray machine came to Nyasaland to the D.G.M. Hospital, donated by the Scottish Sunday Schools. Within a few years Zomba and Blantyre also acquired them.

In the early 1930s, two medical officers with additional surgical qualifications came to Nyasaland. Dr.C.H. Howat F.R.C.S.(Edin) in Fort Johnston Hospital carried out 259 operations, 158 under general anaesthetic, 101 under local. He was pleasantly surprised by the lack of commoner complications seen in Britain: these were fever, postoperative infections, vomiting, and chest problems. He attributed this to the fact that the Nyasaland patients would not stay in bed (which was insisted on in Europe at that time), and kept moving about. We now know early mobilization is important after any operation.

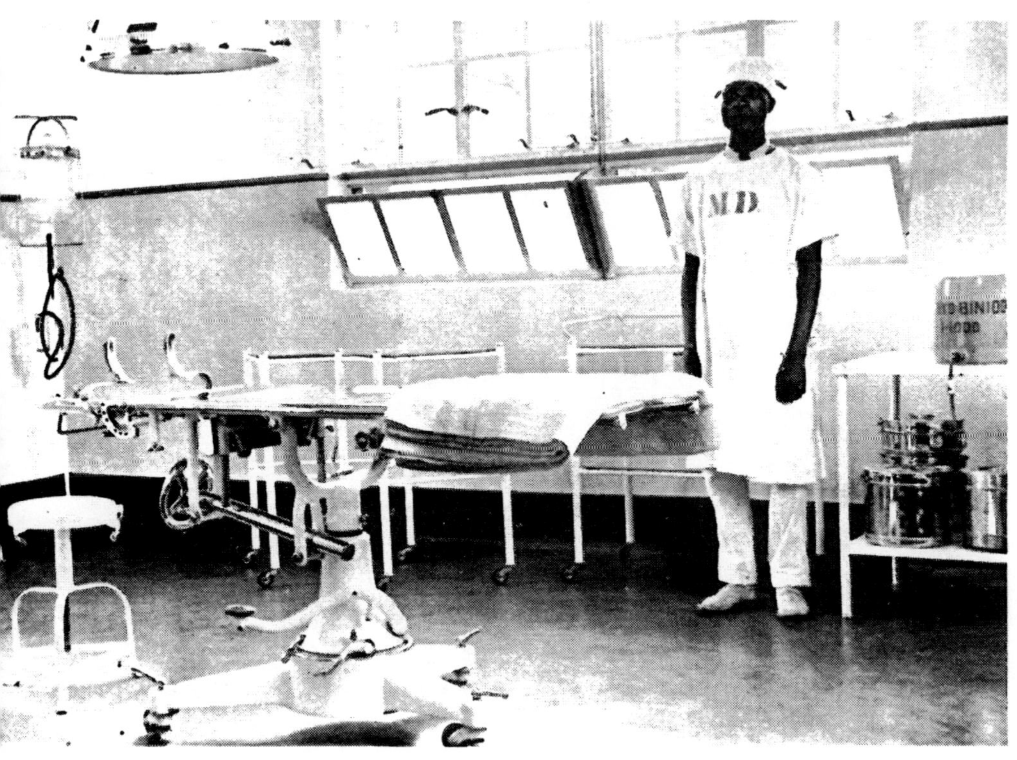

1935 Operating Theatre, African Hospital, Zomba

Dr.H.D. Cronyn F.R.C.S.(Edin) took a special interest in the use of Spinal Anaesthesia and also did three Caesarian operations (removing the baby through an operation in the abdomen) in 1936, surprisingly this is the first named record we could find of this now very common operation. Blood transfusions were first used on a scientific basis at this time. Blood groups were then labelled 1 - 4, before the ABO system was introduced.

In 1942 the first Surgical Specialist, Mr.M.A.W. Roberts was appointed to Zomba General Hospital. He made regular visits to Blantyre. Over the five year period 1946-51, a 62% increase in surgical work was reported. Since then there has been a steady increase in Surgical and other specialists in the country. At the time of writing, there are nine surgeons and one anaesthetist, six obstetricians, and three ophthalmic surgeons.

Some of the first Malaŵian Surgical Specialists (qualifying in the 1970s) have moved into high administrative posts. Dr.H.M. Ntaba (General Surgeon) is now the Minister of Health. The present Chief of Health Services is Dr.P.C. Chimimba (Dental Surgeon), and a previous Chief Medical Officer was Dr.M.C. Chirambo (Ophthalmic Surgeon). Dr.J.D. Chiphangwi (Obstetrician and Gynaecologist) is the Medical School Project Co-ordinator.

SURGICAL OPERATIONS (Government Hospitals)

1951	Major	Minor	Total
Blantyre	118	565	683
Zomba	333	1214	1547
Lilongwe	84	260	344
Total	535	2039	2574

1989	Surgical		Obstetric			
	Major	Minor	Major	(caesarian)	Minor	Total
Blantyre	1306	2641	1718	(1128)	3130	8795
Zomba	376	1082	893	(716)	746	3097
Lilongwe	1025	3041	1405	(901)	1735	7206
Total	2707	6764	4016	(2745)	5611	19,098

Malaŵian Clinical Officers and Medical Assistants now carry out the bulk of the minor surgery in the country. Dr.E.Blair, an orthopaedic surgeon from Canada, has for the past few years been training Orthopaedic Clinical Officers to manage the many fractures and simpler orthopaedic problems.

The motor car has replaced wild animals as the major cause of injury, but many of today's cases would be familiar to the early pioneers: abscesses, tropical pyomositis, osteomyelitis (infection of bone), hernias, burns and tropical ulcers. Just as with the tumours, there are many differences between surgical conditions in Africa and Europe.

Most Africans have a much more physically active life than Europeans or North Americans. They bear enormous weights on their heads and walk long distances and it might be expected that their joints would wear down, but they do not. Arthritis of the hips and spine is however common in the developed world in people who have a more sedentary life. An acute injury due to carrying heavy weights on the head is however not uncommon in Malaŵi. If the carrier stumbles and falls, he/she may dislocate his neck and often damage the spinal cord, producing paralysis of the arms and legs. This type of injury often has a poor outlook.

Carrying weights on the head, and the differences in diet, as well as lifestyle, explain many of the differences in disease as well as cancers. Malaŵians have a low animal fat, high fibre diet, and Europeans vice versa. Twisting of an elongated colon (volvulus) is common in much of Africa, including Malaŵi, and rare in Europe. In Europe, peritonitis (inflammation of the abdominal cavity) is often secondary to appendicitis or diverticulitis of the colon; these are rare in Malaŵi, and the common cause of peritonitis is perforation of the small intestine due to typhoid, which is not seen in Europe. Perforation of a Duodenal Ulcer (and other complications), is common in both Europe and Malaŵi. This sometimes surprises new

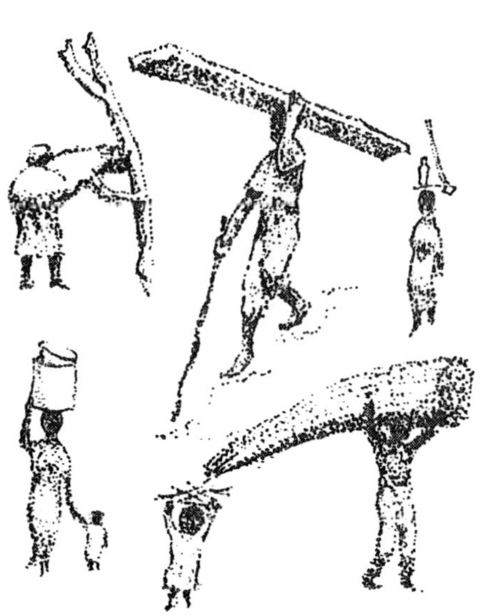

doctors coming into the country. Duodenal ulcer is often linked to stress and a peasant farmer is not seen as one who has much stress. When one thinks a little deeper, it is obvious he has a lot of stress, worry about the crops, getting enough food for his children, and even witchcraft. Arteriosclerosis (hardening of the arteries) is not common in Malaŵi, and Gall Bladder disease, very common in Europe, is very rare in Malaŵi.

Patients respond to surgery well. They are non-complaining, and much younger than the usually 60 -70 year olds in a European ward. The average age of a surgical patient in Malaŵi would be about 22 years.

EYES

One percent of the country's population has severely diminished sight, or is blind. In about half the people, the cause is cataract, or opacity of the lens of the eye.

In the last century, the early doctors (Dr.Prentice among them) were able to improve vision by displacing the opaque lens from the pupil in an operation under local anaesthesia. In the 1920s, an Indian store keeper operated on by Dr.Wigan was so grateful for the restoration of his sight that he gave a large donation to the UMCA. The first mission doctor to specialize in this field was Dr.R.Retief at Nkhoma Hospital in 1928, a tradition carried on in the same hospital today by Dr.C.Blignaut. The first government Ophthalmic specialist (Dr.Peacock) was appointed in 1955 to Blantyre . A succession of Israeli Eye Surgeons came after 1964, and in 1969 special Ophthalmic Medical Assistants training started and the graduates look after eye diseases in the District Hospitals.

There is now the Regional Eye Care Training Programme based in Lilongwe and funded by British Government/ Royal Commonwealth Society for the Blind. Here, Ophthalmic Assistants from surrounding countries are trained.

Cataract surgery remains a major part of the eye work with over 2,000 operations a year performed by the three eye surgeons and three clinical officers. Today the lens is completely removed, and the patient provided with thick spectacles. The Lions' Club set up a spectacle bank, with used glasses from Europe; these are sorted out and given to both cataract operation patients and those with long or short sight. Recently equipment for grinding lenses has been installed.

An ancient major cause of blindness throughout the world is Trachoma, a chronic conjunctivitis which causes scarring and turning inwards of the eyelids. The lashes abrade and scar the cornea, or clear window, of the eye. Surveys in 1967 in Nsanje and other areas showed a high percentage of the population affected, but only a few, serious, complications. Hygienic measures (improving water supplies) and tetracycline ointment have brought the situation under control.

An important cause of blindness in adults is Glaucoma, an increase of pressure within the eye. The Ophthalmic Assistants are able to test for this, and give medical and surgical treatment to prevent deterioration of sight, if it is caught early enough.

In children a major cause of blindness is Keratomalacia, softening and scarring of the cornea. This is due to Vitamin A deficiency in combination with measles and other infections, and is usually seen in malnourished children. Vitamin supplements given early may save the sight. Campaigns for growing leafy vegetables and fruits which contain vitamin A are promoted.

Two mobile eye clinics which have been donated by Blue Peter (a British TV programme) are working here. There are about 350 blind children in special schools, 200 blind people in organized employment, and 60 blind farmers on special estates.

Blue Peter Logo.

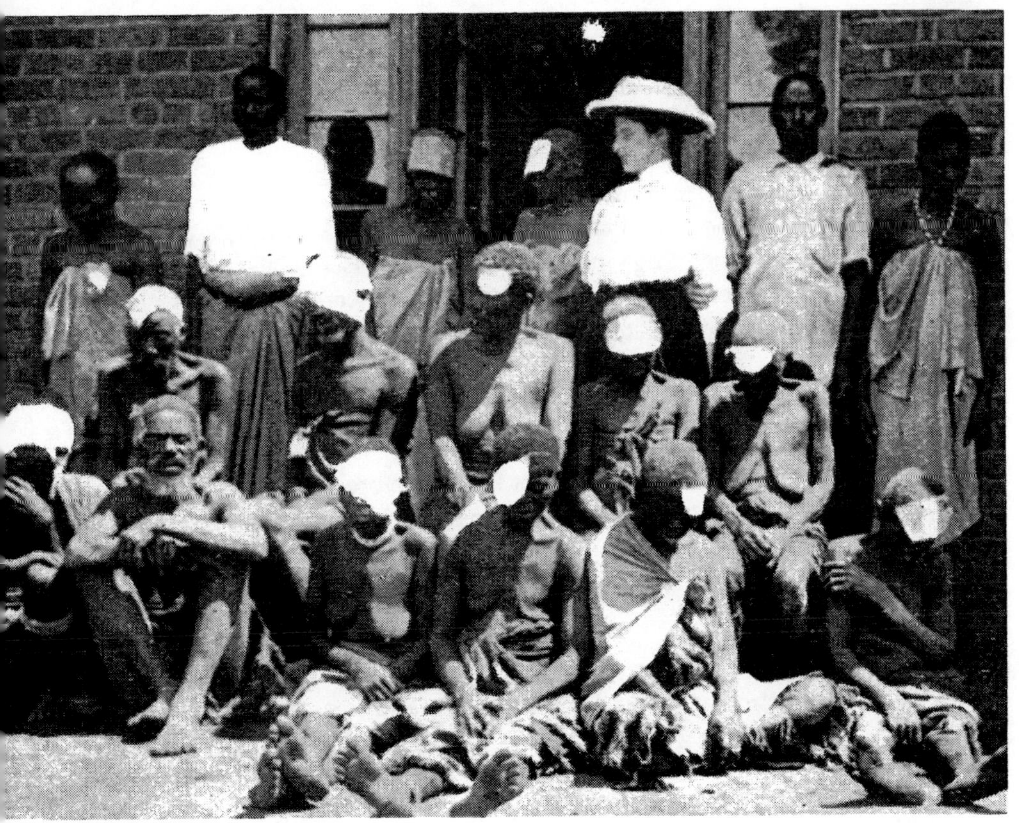

1910 Eye patients with Dr.Mrs.Fraser and two hospital assistants at Loudon (see p.54)

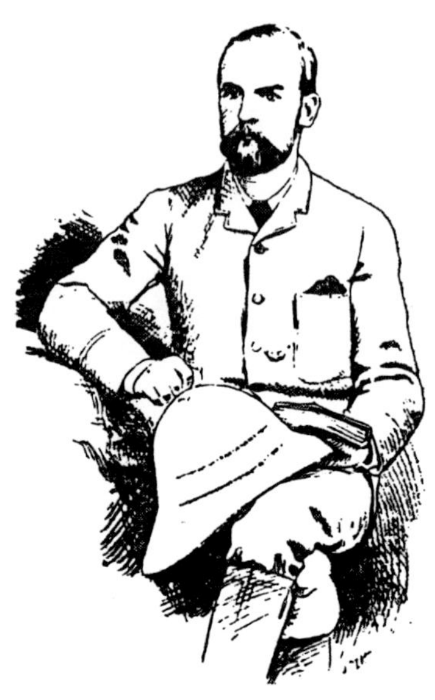

Dr D. Kerr Cross.

In November 1886, David Kerr Cross (M.B. C.M. Aberdeen) brought his Scottish bride, Christina, to the row of little mud houses at Mwiniwanda Mission, situated in the wooded Misuku Hills on the Stevenson road to Tanganyika. It was above a marsh. The ruined cob walls of this Mission, built by James Stewart, can still be seen. The wooden crosses and tombstone beside the murmuring Chirenje stream, at the foot of Chiwuru Mountain, testify the tragedy of malaria at the New Year:

Dr.Cross quietly continued his ministry alone to the diverse tribes in the area of Chief Mwiniwanda, as the whole North End

> *Bakafwakumo*
> *(died)*
> *Christina Kerr Cross 31.12.1886*
> *Hugh Mackintosh 1. 1.1887*

was harassed by Arab slave raiders. The Zanzibar Arab slavers had sent Ruga Ruga men (mercenaries) to assist Chief Mlozi capture victims in the Karonga area. Thousands of slaves were exported from Deep Bay (Chilumba) each year, to go to Zanzibar.

In 1887, the Arabs began a systematic persecution of the Nkonde people: "the Arabs stormed village after village, pillaging and slaughtering without stint; they seized all goods and cattle, the women whom they did not kill, they put in irons, and reserved for a fate still more severe...the Arabs only ceased at sunset, and at night the whole Nkonde Plain was illuminated by fires."(Fotheringham 1887)

In 1888 at Mwiniwanda, Dr. Cross was cut off from all communication with his fellow countrymen. Over and over again he sent messengers to the lakeshore, but they were repeatedly fired at, until the men refused to go. Dr. Cross built a circular stockade of big stones and trees at the top of the hill above the Mission, as a defence against the Arabs. The ruins still stand today. This was called Fort Hill which became the old name of Chitipa District. Fort Hill, with its commanding view across the Nkonde Plain, fell to the Arabs, and Dr.Cross with 200 men, ammunition, and guns, marched to join six other British men in the stockade at Karonga. Led by Monteith

Fotheringham and later with Captain Lugard, they attacked the Arab slavers.

In these forays Dr.Cross was stationed under "the doctor's tree" half a mile away, with all the medical supplies and reserve ammunition. One of his first patients was Fred Moir, who was shot in the arm, and then a little slave boy was injured and Dr.Cross cared for him until he could be returned to his family. Captain Lugard was seriously injured, "he received a bullet which entering his right elbow, tore obliquely across his breast, and finally lodged in his left forearm, where it broke one of his bones." Cross nursed him for several weeks wrapped up in a blanket in a chair.

"The whole Nkonde Plain, over 400 square miles in extent, which was formerly studded with lovely villages teeming with human life, now lay desolate and silent around us." (Fotheringham) After a year's lull, Captain Lugard again attacked Arab stockades in February 1889. Dr.Cross with the baggage and some Nkonde escorts brought up the rear: "he was with us not as a combatant, but as one eager to do his utmost should his medical services be required. We all felt very deeply the warm interest he took in our welfare, both physical and spiritual."

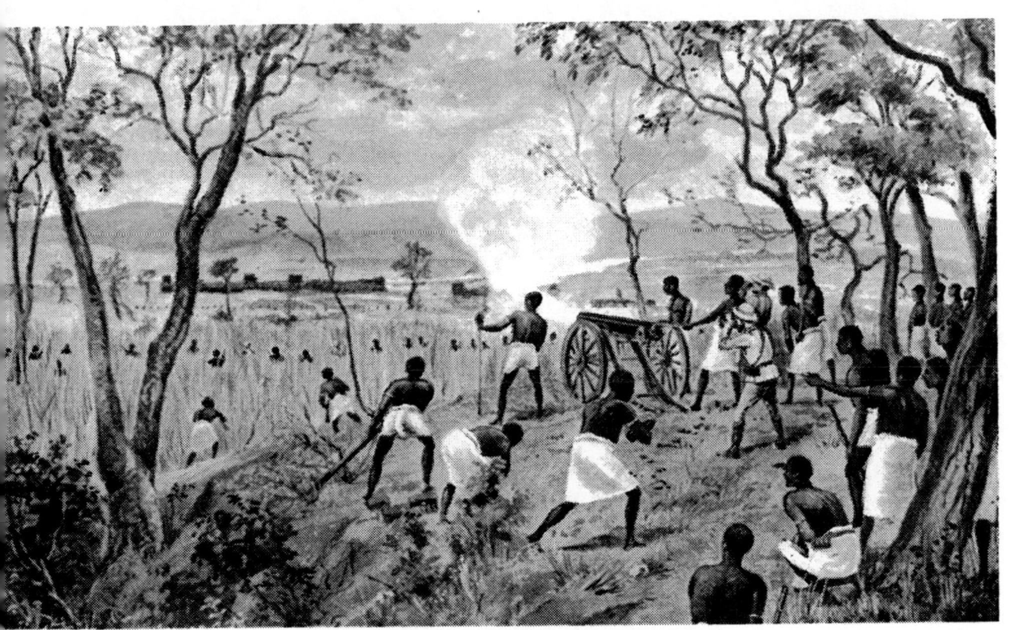

Lugard shelling the slavers stockades

Then smallpox broke out in an Arab camp. "An African woman came to our stockade seeking refuge...she had run away as her people wanted to sell her to the Arabs for cloth. Her husband had died of smallpox and this was the fate reserved for the poor widow. We took her in." (Fotheringham)

In October 1889, Dr.Cross accompanied Consul Harry Johnston's party to negotiate peace with Mlozi, who guaranteed he would not again molest the Nkonde. The British flag was run up in Karonga, and a big fete was held. Dr.Cross stayed a night at Mlozi's stockade on his way back to Mwiniwanda and was "well entertained" by his former enemy. Nkonde huts sprang up everywhere under the shade of the luxuriant bananas, the tinkle of cowbells resounded once more on the plain, and the industry of the people revived. But peace was only temporary.

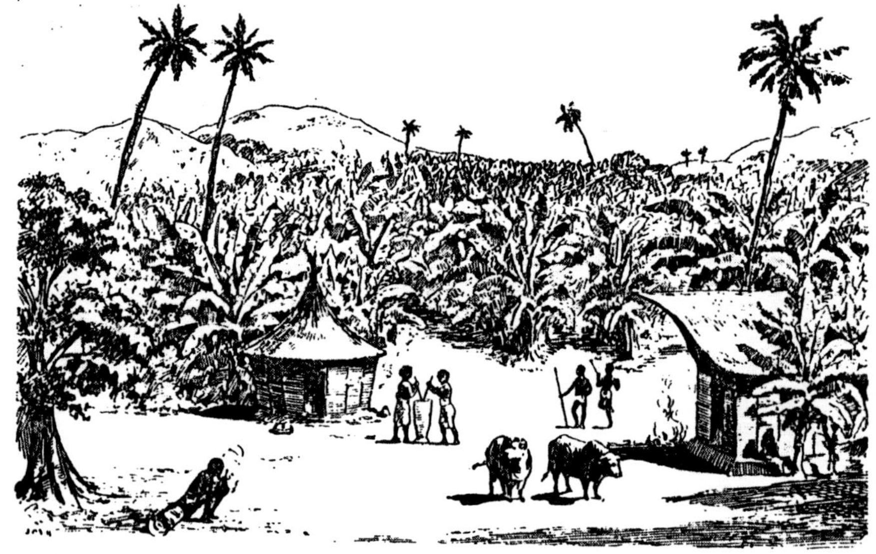

Wankonde Village

David Kerr Cross moved to Karonga in 1889. His calm manner under duress endeared him to all, but the ever present slave trade upset him. Seeing a slave caravan of only 5 boys and 2 girls sitting in their goree sticks at Karonga, he wrote: "poor children, I pitied them with all my heart, and when I saw their upturned eyes and mangled hands, and bruised skinny bodies, and heard the white robed ruffian Arab talk loudly of his property, I felt desperately inclined to break his head...next morning the same caravan came a few miles off their way that they might march past our houses and defy us to touch them."

Then the Ngoni descended from the mountains to attack the Nkonde village of Kayume in 1892, capturing 200 women. Dr.Cross accompanied the Nkonde rescue party, but the Ngoni turned on their captives, killing 45 men and 132 women. Kerr Cross found 47 wounded hiding in the reeds, and wrote "it is heart-rending to see the poor creatures appealing to us."

Dr.Cross quietly established his medical work at Karonga, and he also conducted school lessons under a tree. In 1894 he reported "15 - 35 patients daily, 53 cases of impure diseases, one of mild insanity, 6 major surgical operations under chloroform." Then, "I was called at midnight to see a man two and a half miles away who had been stabbed by an Arab over the right kidney. The patient was removed to my hospital, which is a small African hut, where he made a speedy recovery."

By 1896 his practice had increased to 11,894 outpatients and 53 inpatients, the average per day was over 40 at Karonga. "Many visits were made to villages to attend special cases, and surgical patients were numerous. One man came over 60 miles in September with a diseased arm. He had suffered for fully 5 years, and calmly walking into my dispensary, asked me to cut it off."

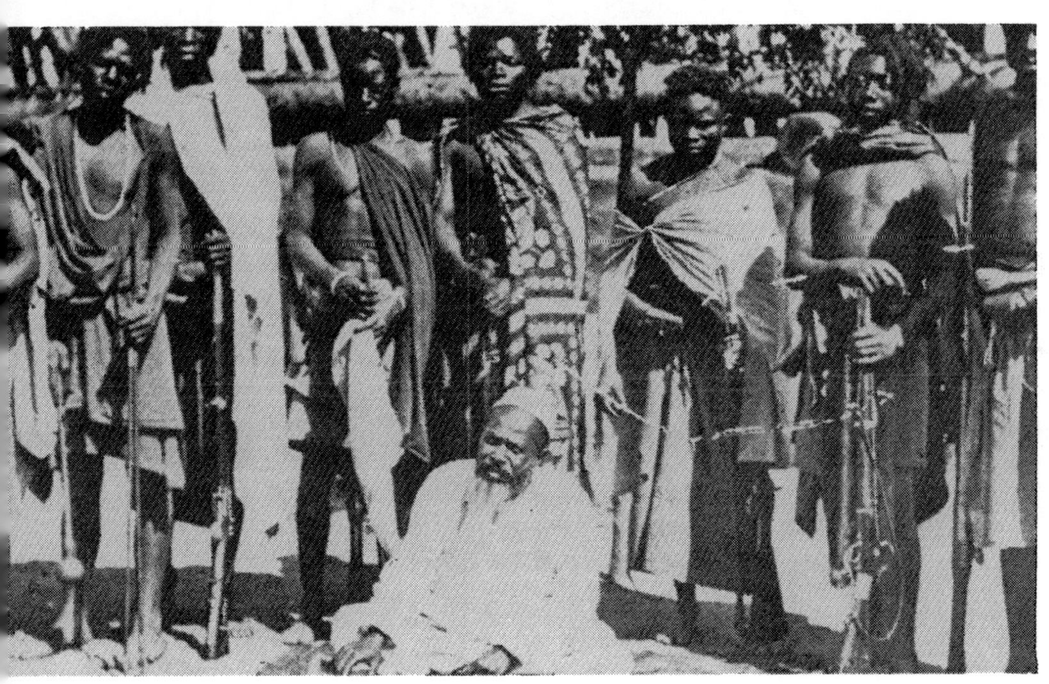

Mlozi and body guards.

The Arabs were finally defeated, and Mlozi was executed in 1896.....''my little hospital was overcrowded with wounded from the late Mpata (Mlozi's village) war. Dr.Poole amputated many shattered limbs. He left 16 cases in my hands.''

David Kerr Cross had a strong sense of justice. In 1895 he reported and had arrested a European who had mistreated an African, and the man was imprisoned for 6 months.

He wrote the first medical report in the Karonga area before he resigned in 1896: ''In my opinion the cases are extremely interesting and offer a splendid field for original work.'' Leprosy was common, syphilis very prevalent (''the Arab disease''), malaria and smallpox were problems, goitre was frequent in Mlozi's village, epilepsy and simple meningitis occurred often, tuberculosis was absent, elephantiasis and filariasis were also seen.

Dr.Kerr Cross joined the Government Medical Services in 1896 and was posted to Zomba and then Blantyre. He left Nyasaland in 1902 for South Africa. His pioneering work among the Nkonde people was the beginning of a long medical tradition at Karonga. His Christian inspiration must have been a humanitarian light shining in the cruel darkness of slavery.

SCOTTISH LADIES

DR. JANE WATERSTON (served 1879)

She was one of the first three British women doctors to qualify in 1879, and immediately came out to work for six months at the Blantyre Mission and at Cape Maclear. She then proceeded to a distinguished Gynaecological career at Cape Town.

DR. MRS. AGNES FRASER *(served 1896-1925)

She was the wife of Donald Fraser, the pioneer missionary at Embangweni. They built the first Loudon hospital there in 1903. She was very interested in obstetrics and ''a few cases came in.'' Not only females wanted her help. In 1908, the last old-style Ngoni Chief, Mzukuzuku, asked to be taken to her ward to be nursed by her, as he lay dying of pneumonia. At his funeral no slave was put to death, as had been the custom until then.

Illus.p.49

8 SMALLPOX

"A mother's son is not her own until he has had the smallpox" English proverb

"Smallpox has marked many" Kirk noted in 1859. Today, young pockmarked faces are not seen. This is because: the disease only affected humans, there was no carrier state, the virus only lives a short time outside the body, and there has been an effective vaccine and campaign of eradication.

Vaccination had been known since 1798 when Dr.Edward Jenner in England had shown that inoculation with cowpox gave protection. Livingstone had cowpox lymph with him in 1859, and he attempted unsuccessfully to propagate and produce more lymph from a cow, in the Zambesi Valley.

The early doctors recorded the local traditional practice of inoculation of children in a smallpox epidemic in the Shire Valley. Material from an infected person was scratched on the web between the thumb and the index finger. This could be dangerous, but if it took, and the patient survived, it would produce lifelong immunity from subsequent epidemics. Epidemics were known and feared by everyone in Nyasaland.They came in two main forms, a milder type and a major type with a 20% mortality.

On August 15th 1890, the White Father noted "Smallpox is raging at Mponda's. Prima, the little girl we bought has been struck down by it. She keeps wailing pitifully to everyone, "ndui, ndui." Perhaps it won't be severe. The father superior vaccinated Brother Antoine and our companion Dominique this morning. Unfortunately our vaccine looked as if it had gone off in the phial."

In 1899 in the Karonga region, during the slave wars, Monteith Fotheringham was suspicious of women from the Arab camps (under Mlozi) who tried to defect to him. He knew smallpox was rife there and suspected they were sent to spread the disease to his soldiers laying siege to the Arabs. Smallpox eventually spread to the Nkonde who were with him. Dr.Kerr Cross was able to isolate patients in a separate hospital and contain the epidemic. He obtained lymph and vaccinated hundreds of Nkonde.

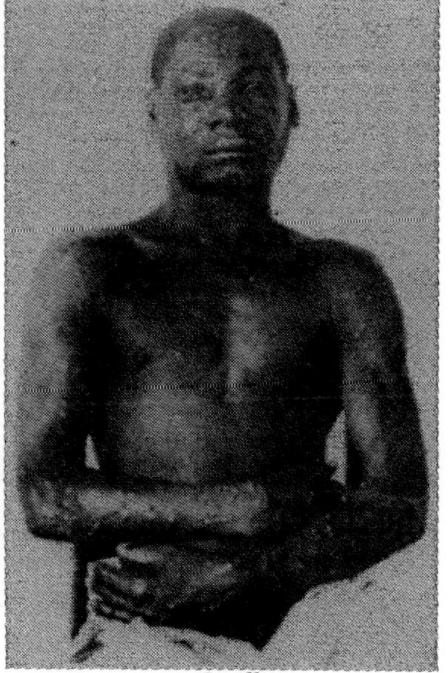

Smallpox

Few years were free of outbreaks however. Vaccine was obtained from Durban in 1891 and 1899. In this last outbreak near Blantyre, Dr.MacVicar was remembered for his services. Although most of his labourers were attacked by smallpox, he vaccinated practically the whole of the population and all those on the Mandala Estate. Nevertheless, in the next year 600 deaths were recorded from the disease in Mulanje and Zomba.

In 1903 "smallpox has been lingering about, Chisangani, Chipaika, and Chintechi, for many months and since the hot weather set in, it seems to be spreading. An elderly man took the disease and went to live in the bush as is usual in most cases of smallpox. It is said that none of his friends would go out to attend him and he died alone." (Bandawe Mission Report).

Many tribes (Ngoni, Tumbuka, Tonga, and Chewa) shared a common belief that those with good moral tone would recover if smitten by smallpox: "whereas on the other hand, if the village does not possess a good moral tone but is given to adultery and other sins, the smitten ones will die both young and old." (Kerr Cross 1895) There was also a local foregoing of funeral feasts at the time of epidemics to prevent spread of the disease.

One result of epidemics was blindness due to corneal ulceration and this led Dr.Howard to set up the blind school in Nkhota Kota in 1904. Systematic vaccination was then started by Government, and £200 a year was set aside for native vaccinators and £100 for lymph. In 1908 a compulsory Vaccination Bill was passed.

The next year, Dr.Prentice at Kasungu was worried about the effects of the lymph he had. "Smallpox outbreaks spread from central Ngoniland...available lymph supply was untrustworthy. I feared the worst. However I vaccinated every person in the village with the exception of a leper and the few natives who had been rendered immune by a previous attack. With the help of a policeman, we tried to isolate a stricken village. When a week, then ten days, passed without any signs of the vaccine having taken, we feared the worst and looked anxiously for fresh supplies of lymph in response to telegraphs and letters. On sabbath evening a fortnight after the people had been vaccinated, I visited the village and examined a suspected case and to my delight found a vesicle on the woman's arm. In a little while, using an ordinary needle, arm after arm was brought into contact with the lymph which oozed from the successful pock. All huts destroyed and the patients moved!"

Public health measures were starting to contain outbreaks. In 1911 there were

78 cases (with 15 deaths) in 6 widely separated localities, but without further spread. Two years later, 143,522 vaccinations were done; but there were outbreaks in Lilongwe (2,786 cases, 864 deaths) and Dowa (767 cases and 77 deaths).This was the first outbreak in Dowa for 6 years. In the same year, 1913, Dr.Davey carried out a survey (basically for sleeping sickness) of nearly 6,000 people in the Dedza area. He found 95% of adults and 9% of children had signs of past smallpox, and he also noted local traditional inoculation of small children.

By 1920, Mr.J.de Meza, a vet, was producing lymph at Zomba from cows. Five years later however doubts on the efficiency of the vaccination campaigns were expressed: 80,699 were vaccinated, 26,973 successful, 28,370 failed (others modified or not seen). "As present carried out, this work can only be regarded as most unsatisfactory. Any medical officer who checks the returns submitted by the native vaccinators will realize that supervision is very important. The figures give a false sense of security as regards the protection afforded the natives against smallpox. The amount of money devoted to vaccination is inadequate, considering the size of the population."

Epidemics continued; in 1930 4,661 cases were reported from Dowa, Mombera, Mzimba, and Lilongwe, with 211 deaths. Ten years later it was feared that a mild outbreak (74 cases with 3 deaths) in the Yao areas might interfere with army recruitment, but an active vaccination campaign brought it under control. 237,048 people were vaccinated. No less than 10 litres of calf lymph were produced in 1947.

Relentlessly the epidemics continued. In 1949 there were several related to the famine in the south, with people migrating to the central regions, and the consequent crowding and decreased resistance. Lilongwe had 199 cases with 49 deaths. The pathologist retired in this year, and lymph production ceased, but there were adequate stored stocks. 740,297 vaccinations were carried out.

"The pestilence raged with virulence, we had not the staff to man the camps in the bush. When the terror died away, they brought in the maimed who were generally children with abscesses with deep pustules, some were blind and all needed a long convalescence with good food."(Nurse at Malosa)

In the 1950s the number of reported cases steadily decreased, (1950:295 cases, 1951:122 cases, 1952:9 cases, 1953:6 cases). In 1955 there were no deaths out of 28 cases and 1,250,000 doses of lymph were produced at Zomba.

There were problems vaccinating: "Knowing that the confirmation of a case would necessitate the closure of a village, it was largely a battle of wits to prevent concealment. For example, a pre-dawn raid of one village revealed that cases were being hidden in the bush from sunrise to sundown. Unfortunately this village had 75% of huts infected." (1949 Health Inspector) In 1956 in Kasungu, women and children would hide in the bush when the vaccinators arrived. In 1960, the Anti-Federation political opposition led to a temporary restriction of vaccinations. There was an outbreak of the disease in the Central Region, and the former Lilongwe Brick and Tile works, 5 miles from the town, was taken over as an isolation hospital. In a five month review period there were 620 cases with 95 deaths. The hospital was closed in 1962 after treating 1,488 cases with 161 deaths.

Small epidemics continued until 1971 when the last nine cases of this disease were reported in Malaŵi. Vaccination continued but by 1977 the last case of smallpox in the world was reported from Mogadishu by the WHO (World Health Organization). A major scourge of mankind had been eliminated.

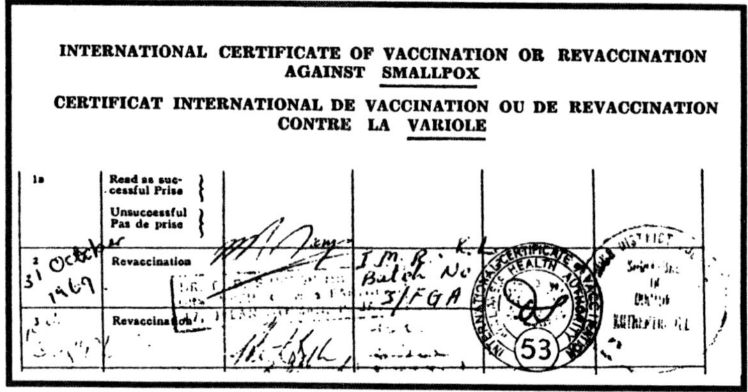

No longer needed

9 THE UNIVERSITIES MISSION

After twenty two years, this Mission returned to Lake Nyasa in 1885 with a centre on Likoma Island. In time it extended medical services to the Yao peoples of the south and eastern sides of the Lake, and also at Nkhota Kota. This area was then harassed by the violence of the slave trade, and witchcraft, similar to that of old Europe, held sway.

The first doctor, Rev.Dr. J. E. Hine, of Oxford University, wrote in 1889 "Three or four women were burnt alive at Chipyela, close to Likoma Mission Station. Maples had done all he could to prevent it...the tragedy took place the night before I arrived." Dr.Hine was invalided home with malaria after a few months. He later returned as Bishop.

Not until 1899 could a permanent doctor be recruited. The lack of doctors in this Mission limited the medical work. In 1906 the Mission reported "there is only one doctor in the diocese; two thirds of the time a nurse has to run hospitals on her own, and be prepared for any emergency." In hospitals without doctors, the health of the Mission staff was at risk, serious injuries needing emergency surgery (which so often came in) could not be adequately treated, diagnoses of disease would have been missed, and policies to observe and control disease could not be made. Without a resident doctor, the local medical staff could only be taught some routine procedures.

DR. ROBERT HOWARD (served 1899-1909)*

As soon as Dr.Robert Howard M.D. B.Ch.(Oxon) arrived, he wrote a report on the health of the Mission staff. In the previous six years, twelve had died and six were invalided home. He recommended proper brick houses, mosquito nets, fumigation of houses, destruction of mosquito larvae, wearing socks after dark, and regular quinine doses. Mission staff health at once improved greatly.

Dr.Howard realised that more hospitals must be built if medical services were to reach the people. When the new Cathedral at Likoma Island was completed in 1905, he immediately converted the old church into a hospital. He sent his butterfly collection to England to be sold, and he launched the "Hospital

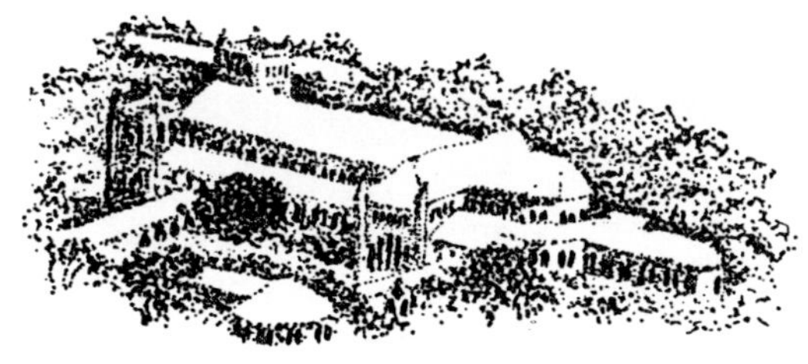

Likoma Cathedral

** Illus. inside front cover*

Mat Fund" in Britain. A subscription of £3 would support one hospital mat/bed for a year in Nyasaland.

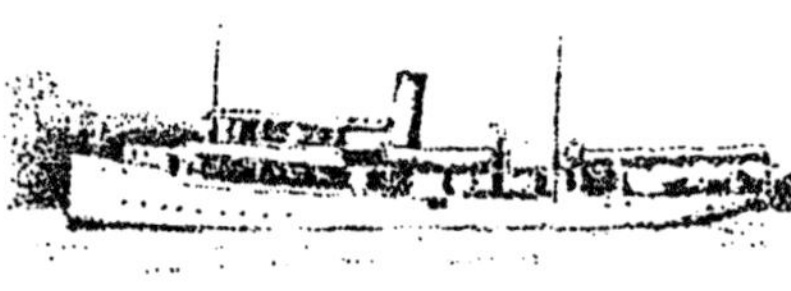

The Chauncy Maples

As a versatile builder, carpenter, harbour master, store keeper, and gardener, Dr.Howard built Nkhota Kota hospital (1902), and Malindi and Mtonya hospitals (1908). The mission steamer **Chauncy Maples** visited lakeshore villages and transported patients to hospital when necessary, Howard commented "a month in hospital transforms a crawling skeleton with ulcers into a fat cheerful person."

Nurse Kathleen Mintner, who later married Dr.Howard, described Nkhota Kota just after the huge slave trade had been suppressed: "When I first arrived in 1899, it was many months before anyone would come for treatment. The people were suspicious. It was incomprehensible to them that an outsider should wish to help the sick... as time went on, they became less suspicious and came with sores and minor ailments...when attendance at dispensaries became fairly numerous, we could open a hospital, but this must be a local mud building. An elaborate brick building at this stage would remain permanently empty."

She gave an interesting side light on slavery: "My first Nkhota Kota patient was a slave wife, who had fallen in the fire and burnt her arms and knees badly. Her husband simply went off on a journey, and abandoned her, locked out of the house. When I found her, she had been lying there for five days, keeping herself alive by eating a stick of raw cassava, and drinking some stale water. No one around would help her."

"The first Mohammedan patient stood some distance off, explained his illness through the mouth of his slaves, who then took the medicine to their master, having first tasted it to be sure it was not poison."

Local self help supported these hospitals,"Every patient brings an offering of food or money, and all who are able help in preparing food and gardening...cotton trees at Nkhota Kota produce excellent down which is splendid for stuffing pillows. Peter (a patient) could pick over this down, make covers for it, and turn out charming cushions."

Kapok Tree.
Unripe pods

Another Nkhota Kota patient "Neema, our one-legged cook, was the first African here to wear a wooden leg. It is wonderful how active she is, how well she does her work, cooking for the men and women and keeping the kitchen clean."

A Nkhota Kota teacher with diphtheria, fortunate enough to be stricken when Dr.Howard was there, had a tracheostomy to allow him to breathe, "by the light of two lamps, his poor wife sitting on the floor with her back to the bed, dreading that each moment would be his last."

He treated many animal injuries: "The wild beasts that cause most injuries are lions, leopards, hyenas, crocodiles, and hippopotami. In 1908-9, we have had a lot of leopard bites with wounds on the head and body; a leopard seems to spring for the throat."

"One man came to us whose arm had been completely bitten off by a hippo. His friends had put on a tourniquet to stop the bleeding, and he walked over 30 miles to the Mission, taking three days over the journey. Though apparently Mr.Hippo had not lately cleaned his teeth, he had done his amputation very cleverly. In spite of acute inflammation, the wound healed up after a time, and to look at the stump, you might have thought it was the work of a clever surgeon!"

The problems of the early Missions were considerable as told in this report from Chigaru in 1908: "The day after I arrived, it rained heavily, until there was not a dry square yard in the house, the roof leaked so badly. However with the help of the boys, my things were hurried over to the teacher's house. I slept there with the teacher and all his hens. The hens cackled and gurgled all night round my net, perhaps because I had roused them up. Have you ever slept in a house with many chickens round you? I turned up the lamp to see if they really were asleep and they were, with their heads under their wings, some standing on one leg and some on two."

Dr.Howard realised the urgent need to train African staff. "In the early days none of the scholars wanted to be Dawa (medicine) Boys. They disliked touching ulcers. In 1900 Dr.Howard asked Edward Nemeleyani to take up this work. At first he refused, and later on accepted. The doctor was pleased and started to teach him. Then the rest of the boys

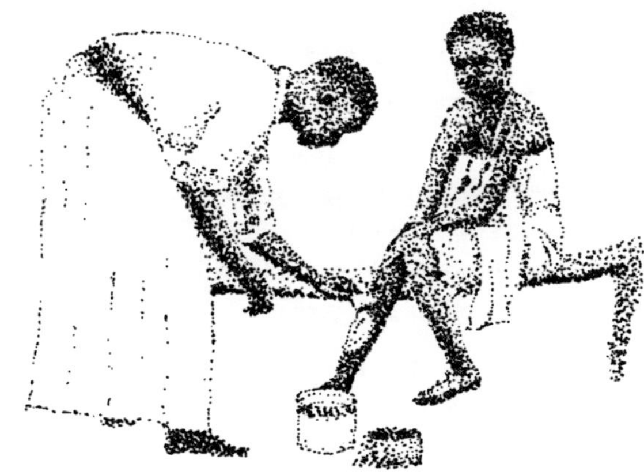

Dressing ulcers (from an old photo).

became angry and laughed at him. They called him 'touch ulcers'...Edward bore it with a humble steadfastness that gradually wore away opposition." Mr.Nemeleyani worked as a Medical Assistant for 48 years at Likoma and Matope.

European medicine and medical methods were still regarded with deep suspicion by African public opinion, but Raphael Mbwana also came to learn. "Raphael is clever, quick, and methodical, he always keeps his head and rises to an emergency. He is excellent during operations" wrote Dr.Howard. At Malindi "Guy Matekwe is an old patient operated on by Dr.Hine. He is quite crippled from burn contractures...he seems really keen on his work and asked to take his physiology books home for the holidays." "Ambrose Masiye and Manfred were also being trained as Dispensary Assistants, surveying all the outpatients each morning and selecting those who should be referred to the hospital," at Nkhota Kota.

In 1905, a gift of Braille books enabled the Mission to start the first Blind School in Nyasaland at Nkhota Kota, with 16 pupils. "Enquiries were diligently made for blind folk, and with much persuasion, several were prevailed upon to leave their homes. They do manual work making mats, brushes, baskets, and string, in the mornings, and they learn Braille in the afternoon. When they sing in Church they nearly raise the roof."
The U.M.C.A. celibacy rules obliged Dr.Howard to leave when he married Nurse Mintner in 1909.

DR. WILLIAM WIGAN (served 1911-47)

Dr.William C. Wigan (from Bart's Hospital,London) came to Likoma Island, to serve for 35 years, which included the impoverished times of two World Wars.

In 1914, an appeal from Likoma Mission to Britain read: "I am generally in the last gasp for old linen before the next lot comes. At the present time our numbers in the Dispensary run up to 200 - 300 daily. Will our

Dr. Wigan

readers please send some? The War Office forbids the export of bandages, therefore the demand for all sorts of white rags suitable for dressing wounds (old table cloths, cotton sheets etc.) is greater than ever before."

In this deprivation, Dr.Wigan embarked on major surgery. He managed the first ever surgical/obstetric patient at Nkhota Kota Hospital: "We had an interesting maternity case in a Mohammedan family...it was due to much tact on Nurse Burridge's part that I was allowed to operate and give chloroform. "At Likoma Hospital: "One little Wampoto girl with legs deformed by rickets, has had two operations with a view to strengthening them and helping her to walk. Operations average two a week under anaesthesia. The new operating theatre is a boon, with space, air, and good light. It was first a vestry, then a house, then a store, and now an operating room."

"At Nkhota Kota we brought one woman requiring (and begging for) an amputation of her arm. At Mponda's, I removed a large piece of dead bone from a boy's heel. We get a lot of such cases here, owing to early neglect of wounds and ulcers." Yet Dr.Wigan had to use local raw cotton with beeswax or palm oil to dress ulcers. His ability to supply care in the most limited situations was remarkable. Local cotton was boiled with soda although the results were not very absorbent or satisfactory. He mentioned that cases of yaws, syphilis, malaria, bilharzia, hookworm, and tick fever, were common. He treated yaws with arsenic injections, and bilharzia with injections of sodium antimony tartrate.

After hostilities began in 1914, Dr.Wigan continued to supply care to the lepers on Lundu Island (German territory), whilst the Germans supplied food, an impressive example of enemy co-operation. Despite the war, he improved the course for training Medical Assistants, writing Yao and Chewa physiology books.

In 1917, he enlisted in the King's African Rifles, returning to increased problems in the Universities' Mission in 1919. Not only was financial aid from Europe greatly reduced, but the Mission was asked to take over three hospitals abandoned by the Germans in Tanganyika.

There was a bad famine in 1922, and wild animals became hungry too: "People are swarming here for food, and besides this, lions are devouring people, 16 at Lungwesi, 6 at Msisi, and 13 at Luchilongo." By 1923 he noted "we have had over 1,000 inpatients and more than 100,000 outpatients in the Mission Stations."

1921 Likoma Island	
431 patients	
Ulcers	
Abscesses	60%
Injuries	
Worms	10%
Yaws	7%
Bilharzia	5.5%

At Likoma a monthly 2p ticket was charged for outpatient treatment. At Mponda's there was no ticket, but offerings of food were requested: "but the offering we like best of all is for them to go to their villages and make it possible for us to build a school there and start work. This does happen over and over again."

The first high powered microscope at Likoma in 1925 made diagnosis easier. Bilharzia and hookworm eggs could easily be seen, and Dr.Wigan instructed his medical assistants that "all blood specimens for malaria, tick fever, and tubercle or leprosy bacilli, must be sent to my oil immersion microscope at Likoma or to the Government Medical Officer at Fort Johnston."

He pioneered improved care for leprosy patients with leper wards at Likoma, Malosa, Malindi, and Mponda's stations, so as to keep infectious patients away from the villages. By 1930 his work had spread to 9 hospitals reaching 381 villages, and he had a staff of 18 nurses and 25 Dawa boys (Dressers) in training. They cared for 2,297 in-patients, and 218,484 outpatients.

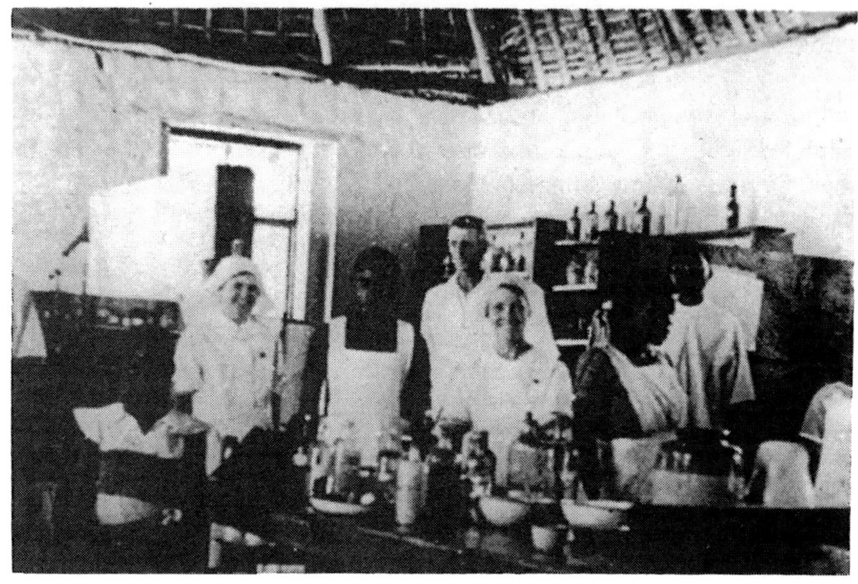

Dr. Wigan and staff in the pharmacy

The Universities' Mission hospitals were depicted in 1930: "Picture a long mud building, with a roof of poles and midribs of large palm leaves, tied together with strips of bark, topped with grass thatch. There are few windows. Inside the walls are white with alabastine which deters ants...round the room are beds and the floor space is occupied by mats made of palm leaf. There is an open fireplace at one end. All medicines and dressings are carried to the ward from the dispensary. Thanks to Dr.Wigan and our supporters at home, we are well supplied with the latest remedies and some very up to date apparatus. A bad case of mauling by a lion or a crocodile is fixed up by Carrel tubes and dressed up in a style you would see in a London surgical ward. A nurse who joined us two years ago was very struck by the fact that the treatment was so up to date."

"An operation room is attached to each of our Mission hospitals. The appointments are simple but adequate. Last year a high pressure sterilizer was added to two of our stations. This sterilizing is done over a wood fire in the open, and by pulling out the burning sticks when the pressure is too high, or adding wood when it is too low, we achieve in a small way what is done with gas or electricity at home."

The patients do not lie in bed or on their mats: all who can crawl go out into the sun, the utterly helpless are carried out ...by Lake Nyasa one can always eat fish, it is so simple, you scrape it and toast it on a stick over the ward fire. In the late afternoon, the patients sit outside with their relatives who come into hospital with them to look after them. In the centre is the fire and the large cooking pot with nsima for 40 patients. At last it is cooked, grace is said. The sun is setting low, the hospital chickens are flying into the one tree where they sleep. The patients are all sitting on the ground eating their nsima, and there we say goodbye."

In his time, Dr.Wigan built wards at Linti, Manda, Milo, (Tanganyika), Likoma Island, Malosa, Malindi, Mponda's, and Matope. The work was mainly confined to surgery and medicine. Only a few mothers wanted help in childbirth.

In 1939 the Bishop appealed: "we need a second doctor to help Dr.Wigan in the exacting work of the medical supervision of the hospitals, dispensaries, and staff, of 11 Stations, scattered in a line of 400 miles from Matope to Milo. Dr.Wigan has been coping with this gigantic task for over 25 years, with an energy that seems providentially to increase with the amount of work to be done. He spends nine months of the year travelling, only staying sometimes for a few days in his house at Likoma."

Dr.Wigan worked on until 1947, when he retired aged 70. The Bishop wrote "I mention his unerring and patient skill as a doctor and a surgeon; the high standard, personal and professional that he has set himself and demanded of all his staff, and his scrupulous financial economy."

The influence of Dr.Howard and Dr.Wigan, who were mindful of the Great Physician, spread far beyond their own patients. Slowly thousands of people around the Lake came to understand the value of Christian humanitarian attitudes and of modern scientific medicine. "We Africans are grateful to our beloved physician for his zealous work, and because of all the African staff he has trained. Dr.Wigan loved and walked with Our Lord."

Today the UMCA hospitals are at Malosa (Likwenu), Nkhota Kota, and Malindi, with a full staff headed by a Doctor or Senior Clinical Officer.

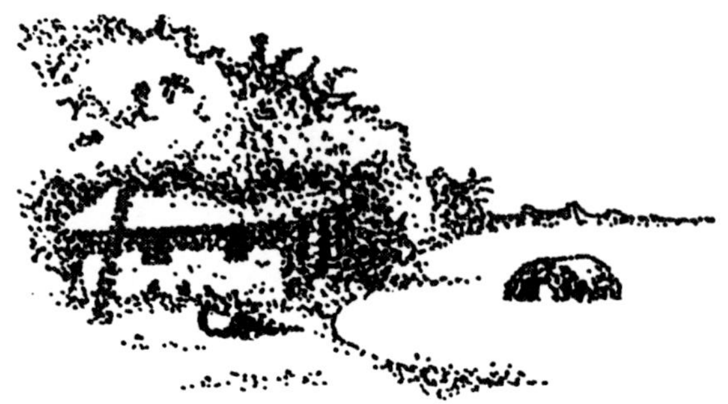

Malindi today. The old boiler of the Chancy Maples lies in the lake near the engineering workshop that used to service Lake steamers

Girl recovering from crocodile wounds

A six-year-old girl, Dalitso ████, is recovering in Nkhotakota Hospital from wounds she sustained in a crocodile attack at Tambala Village near the *boma* on January 10.

Dalitso's father, Mr. ████████, said that he and two friends rushed to the scene of attack in Cham'dilo Stream to rescue the girl from the crocodile's jaws after they heard her crying for help.

Dalitso sustained deep wounds on both thighs and at the back.

A duty nurse at the hospital, Miss Paulina ████, said that the girl arrived in a very weak state, but her condition improved tremendously after receiving five pints of intravenous fluids.

An official from the district's Parks and Wildlife Office said that two hunters had been sent to the area to shoot the crocodile, but the marauding reptile was still at large. — Mana

Daily Times 16.1.1992

Even in the rural Mission Hospitals the motor car has replaced animals as the major cause of severe injury. There are still a significant number of crocodile and hippopotomus attacks.

Dogs are required to be vaccinated against rabies. Bites by domestic and wild rabid animals occur uncommonly but when the animal is suspect anti rabies vaccine must be given.

Puff adder bites on bare feet are the commonest snake bite, usually not severe. Snakes are shy animals and are rarely encountered by visitors even in the bush.

PLAGUE

"We are dying in our village, investigate, come immediately".

This was a telegram to Dr.Frank Innes at Livingstonia, from Karonga. He arrived on January 26th 1917 and found six people had already died. A fatal rat illness had preceded the human cases. On February 10th his microscope arrived "there were the short, round ended, various sized, bipolar staining, bacilli pestis, of bubonic plague." By March, 19 out of 32 cases had died (a 59% mortality). Dr.Prentice later telegraphed to say he had found 2 cases at New Langenburg (Tanganyika) confirmed by military medical officers.

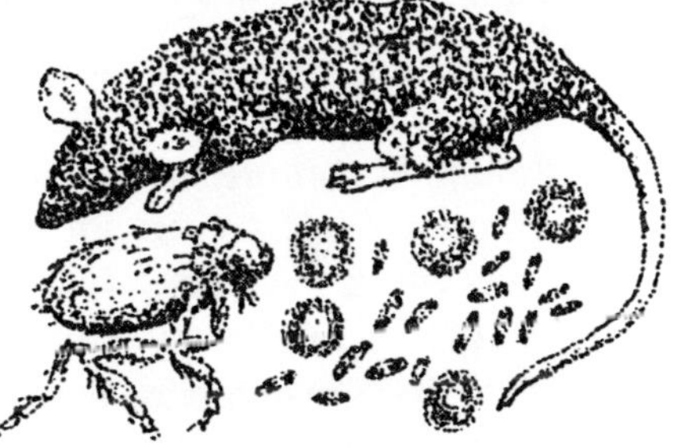

This was the first recorded introduction into Central Africa of the Plague. The disease is sufficiently distinctive to be recognized from ancient writings; there are bubos (swollen lymph nodes), black patches of skin(the Black Death), and congestion of the lungs(in pneumonic form).

320 BC "Then the Lord laid a heavy hand on the people of Ashod. He threw them into distress and plagued them with tumours (bubos) and the land swarmed with rats." I Samuel 5/6.

Rat, flea and plague bacteria among red blood cells (magnified).

It has a fearsome reputation for causing death; in 542 A.D. about 10,000 people a day had died of plague in Constantinople. The Black Death in the 14th and 17th Centuries decimated populations in Europe and resulted in far reaching social changes. The global epidemic that arrived in Central Africa had started in China in 1894. There Yersin and Kitasato had identified a bacterial cause. There is an animal reservoir in rodents, and the bacillus is spread by fleas. The authorities were worried when plague reached South Africa, Chinde and Zanzibar in 1905. Chinde (Mozambique) at the mouth of the Zambesi, was the port of entry to British Central Africa, and special measures were taken to prevent spread.

The disease broke out in Karonga in 1916 with 13 cases reported. Energetic efforts to catch rats were made in 1917 when there were 28 cases. Three million were eventually killed. "Trapping is carried out by small boys, and to some extent by women, who day after day troop in with their catches, and

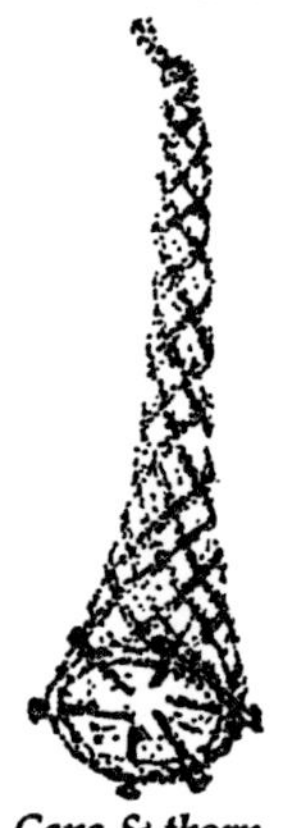

*Cane & thorn
rat trap*

at the end of the month must reap a reward exceeding by far their wildest dreams of wealth.......it was a common sight to see a small boy of about 10 years of age receiving as much as 16-25 shillings." (The rate of pay for an ordinary labourer was then 4-6 shillings a month-Lamborn). Not surprisingly, the purchase of rat tails was later discontinued, and poison was also used.

In 1918, there were only 5 cases of plague, but the local rat population carried the bacillus, and throughout Africa, from time to time, small epidemics occur.

In 1924 there were four fatal cases. Four women who came from the Fort Maguire area at Makanjila's, slept at a village six miles from Fort Johnston on the previous night. One was taken ill during the night, and was carried in to hospital; the other three walked in; all died within 30 hours. Post mortem examination showed the lungs to be congested and haemorrhagic; smears showed bipolar gram negative staining bacilli. The huts where the women had slept were burnt, and patrols posted on the Fort Maguire road. There were no further cases. In 1939 there was a small outbreak at Neno (3 cases),following an outbreak of deaths in rats. In 1956 there were 20 cases with 3 deaths in the Port Herald district. In 1963, there were 30 probable cases with 9 deaths in Ngabu.

There are now effective antibiotics to treat plague. It is not a major health problem in Africa, although there were outbreaks in Mozambique in 1976, and in Kenya in 1978.

THE WILY JIGGER

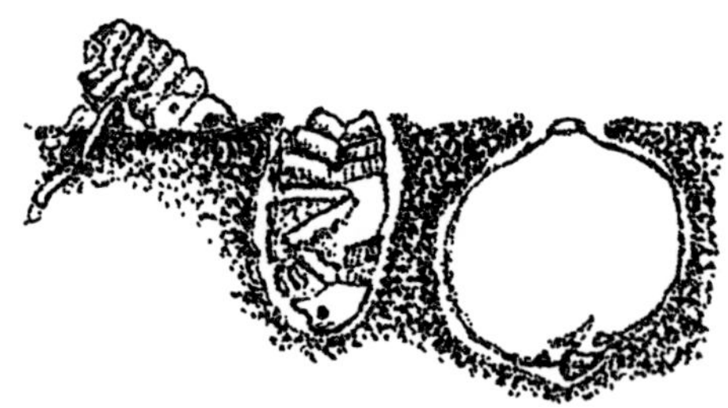

Jigger burrowing into skin.

The Jigger (Matakenya) is a sandflea. The female burrows into the feet around the toes and enlarges to the size of a pea full of eggs which it discharges intermittently. Infections and nasty sores may develop.

The jigger is said to have been brought to West Africa in 1872 in sand ballast from Brazil. The insect seems to have entered Nyasaland at Karonga in 1892, along the slave and trade routes. Dr.Kerr Cross remarked in 1895 at Karonga that up to three and a half years previously, jiggers were unknown along the Lakeshore. He advocated needle removal and the application of carbolic acid, iodoform, and glycerine. "Of a dozen surgical cases of a morning, 11 are likely to be ulcers and of these 10 will probably have a history of Matakenya."

Europeans were not immune: "it was part of one's morning toilet to have jiggers removed from one's feet by African experts." Dr.Laws once removed twelve from his feet, and held school jigger parades. A correspondent (to the Central African Planter in 1896) who left Nyasaland for England some months previously, "writes to say that he actually had the pleasure of extracting a jigger from one of his toes in London. It must have been in his foot during the voyage, that is a period of six weeks."

1906 "Jiggers are the scourge of the Yao Hills and probably medical development there will require a specially constructed Jigger Hospital." "It is quite easy to tell when a person has jiggers. He/she gets a walk characteristic of the complaint." Nurse Mintner.

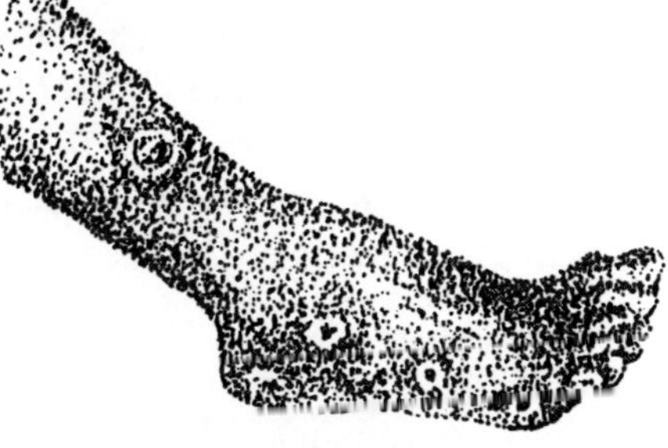

Ulcers due to jiggers.

After the Second World War the new insecticides D.D.T. and gammexane were sprayed around huts to kill ticks, fleas, and mosquitoes. This led to a rapid decrease in jiggers and it is only occasionally seen today.

TICK BORNE RELAPSING FEVER

This disease, with its recurrent bouts of fever and weakness, can be confused with malaria, but the diagnosis can be made by finding the spiral organism in the blood film. It was an endemic problem in the early days and a significant cause of death. Livingstone himself suggested that relapsing fever was transmitted by ticks, but it was Dutton and Todd who proved this in 1905 (they were here on the Sleeping Sickness Commission).

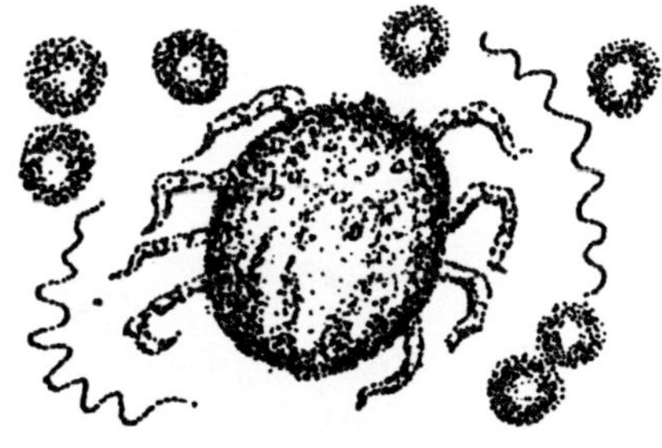

Tick and bacteria among red blood cells (magnified).

In 1909 Mwenzo Mission reported "tick fever less than last year. Three deaths out of 39 cases cause the natives to sleep outside in preference to a 'Nkufu' infested hut." Nkufu or tampan was the tick (O.morbata) that lived in cracks in buildings and transmitted the bacteria. These ticks could not move far and so the disease was one of places and buildings. Indeed it was often the reason for abandoning a hut.

Locals in the area would build up some degree of immunity but newcomers might succumb to the new variety of bacteria. Dr.Ransford recorded that he had met locals, who when they went on ulendo (travelled) would carry their own ticks in little boxes and allow them to bite, to preserve a degree of immunity. As with malaria, and some bacterial and viral infections, the outer coat of the organism may change and defeat the degree of immunity built up by a patient.

In 1913 Dr.Turner at Bandawe wrote "would anyone like to donate some iron bedsteads from home? One is rather smitten with shame when patients complain of the number of biting insects in the wards; and then, when you asked them 'why do you not sleep on the beds rather than on the floor?' say that the things on the beds are worse than on those on the floor!"

There was no specific remedy and no effective easily available insecticides in those days. Most cases came from the Northern and Central Regions, and there were about 80 a year reported, with about a 5% mortality. As with most diseases, this probably grossly underestimated the true prevalence. In 1949, 552 cases were reported with 5 deaths. By this time, Gammexane and D.D.T. (long lasting residual insecticides), had become available, and it was possible to control the ticks. Spraying, and surrounding huts by a ditch filled with sand and insecticide, would protect for up to two years. When penicillin, and later tetracycline, became available, a safe treatment was possible.

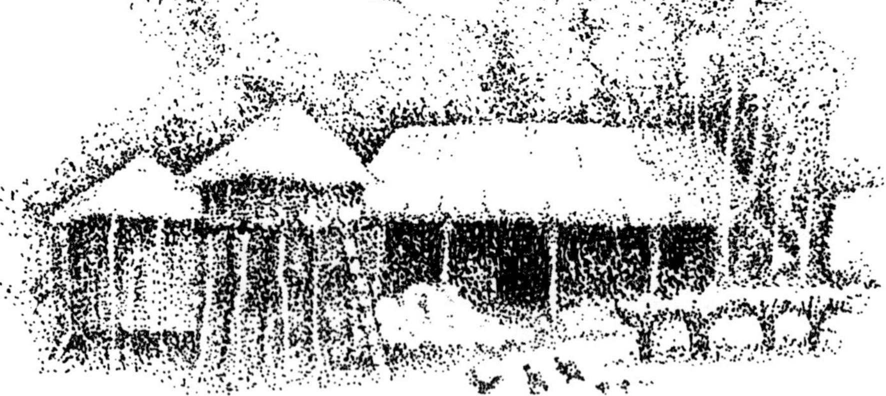

An unchanging scene.Insecticides, when affordable, have however dramatically changed the infestation of homes and crops.

11   DR. and MRS. WALTER ANGUS ELMSLIE
(served 1884-1924)

"My own home, my own wife, are precious to me" Gaelic saying

The Scottish Church sent Dr.Elmslie (M.B. C.M.Aberdeen) to take charge of the Ngoniland Mission in Chief M'mbelwa's Village of Njuyu in 1884. The Ngoni people were Zulus who had left Natal during the cruel 'mfecane' of Chief Chaka in the 1820s. The largest tribal group settled in the northern hills above Lake Nyasa.

Elmslie wrote "The peoples of other tribes were driven to live in

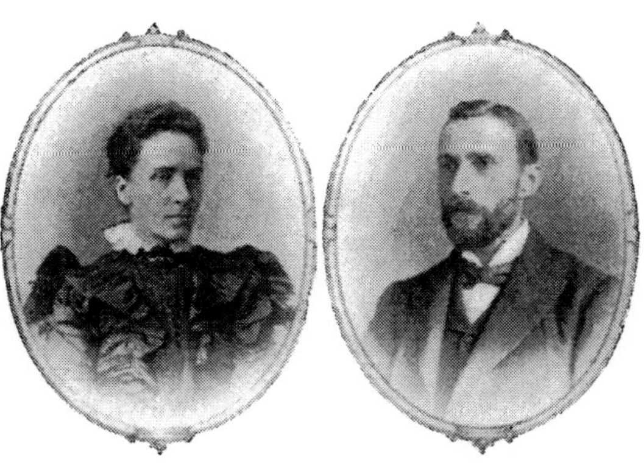

Dr. & Mrs. W. Elmslie

rocky, inaccessible, places, but Ngoniland was then a great expanse of land...dotted over with numerous villages, built without regard to safety from attack, but located where the best gardens and pastures were...here were a people powerful and free." "Removing a village to a new site was a great event. It was a religious occasion. The cattle kraal (fold) was built first in a huge circular area. Then a cow was sacrificed to ancestral spirits and eaten by the people...the huts of the people are built in circles around the cattle kraal, walled off from each other by reed fences, so that each man with his wives'huts and those of his slaves, is a distinct locality. The Chief's hut, with his seraglio and slaves, is opposite the cattle kraal. Inside this kraal all Indabas (tribal discussions) occur and village dances take place."

William Koyi, the fine Zulu missionary from Natal, took Dr.Elmslie to meet Chief M'mbelwa "with his piercing gaze" to ask if he could settle and do medical work there. M'mbelwa replied that the country did not belong to him, but to his people, so if his Indunas (headmen) approved, Elmslie could stay. A week later Dr.Elmslie was summoned to a huge Indaba of hundreds of warriors and Indunas. The day began with fearsome war dancing, in the cattle kraal at Njuyu.

The men said "You have medicines, we hope you will give us medicines to make our slaves obedient, and to quiet our enemies." However they would not allow any teaching. "If we give you our children to teach, your words

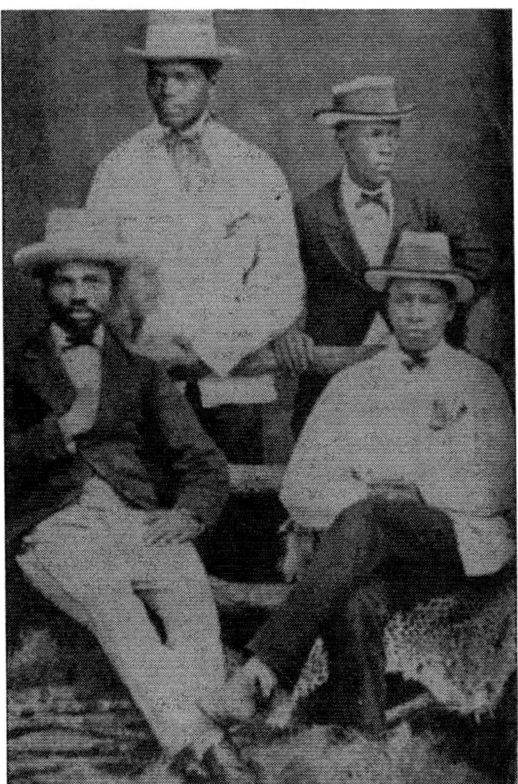

Wiliam Koyi (front left) with the three other Lovedale evangelists. Mopas Ntintili (back left) with Shadrach Nguna who died of TB at Cape Maclear beside him. Isaac Wauchope (front right).

will steal their hearts, they will become cowards, and refuse to fight for us when we are old; and knowing more than we do, they will despise us." Finally Chief M'mbelwa expressed joy that Elmslie was skilled in medicine. He himself was often sick, and there were few old men around, because they had all died young.

Dr.Elmslie noted that he was living at Njuyu on sufferance. The Ngoni did not need his protection, because they were masters of the country for miles around. He wrote "I have seen an Ngoni army, 10,000 strong, go forth in June and not return until September, laden with captured women, slaves, cattle, and ivory, and nearly every man painted in white clay denoting he had killed someone.

"The doctor opened his dispensary in 1884: "at first people came in crowds. Those who were sick expected medicines to keep them well...one of the greatest effects of medical work was that the empiricism of the witch doctors was overthrown; and the people, ignorant and superstitious, were rescued from the bondage of their shrewd incantations...the witch doctors say it is the will of the Spirits that the patients must die"

Elmslie's pioneer colleagues then perished. James Sutherland from Wick, Caithness, who had worked at Njuyu for four years and made the first bricks in Ngoniland, died in 1885. The Ngoni danced their sorrow for the death of Sutherland, and asked if witchcraft had caused his demise. Then George Rollo died a week after arriving at Njuyu on a horse. This horse caused widespread fear. Women believed their babies would be born as monsters.

"After the strain of nursing Mr. Rollo, I was worn out, and I had a sharp attack of fever myself, the result of over anxiety and fatigue. People complained to Chief M'mbelwa of our supposed evil powers: we were accused of all the family disasters, the non-success in battle, the death of cattle, the fleeing of slaves, and the drought."

Then in 1886 came a change. Three sons of a powerful witchdoctor came to Dr.Elmslie for instruction. Chitezi, Mawalera, and Makera, arrived, and "we spent several hours together every evening and they made rapid progress in reading and writing. Chitezi was married, he had been distinguished in several fights, and received commendations for his prowess. Hallowed were those hours in the stillness of the night with these Ngoni young men. It was touching to hear them pray for the enlightenment of their witchdoctor father, for their friends, the Chief, and the Indunas."

Elmslie's reputation was also enhanced when it happened to rain after public prayers for rain. Mawalera Tembo's grandson said in 1990 at Njuyu,"Mawalera told me he was a mouthpiece for Elmslie to the Ngoni people, and advised the tribal Council to accept Christian medicine and teaching. Before the Christians came, the Ngonis were very cruel and warlike. Mawalera asked the chiefs not to attack the Azungus (Europeans), but to welcome the changes they were bringing, and to abandon washing their spears".

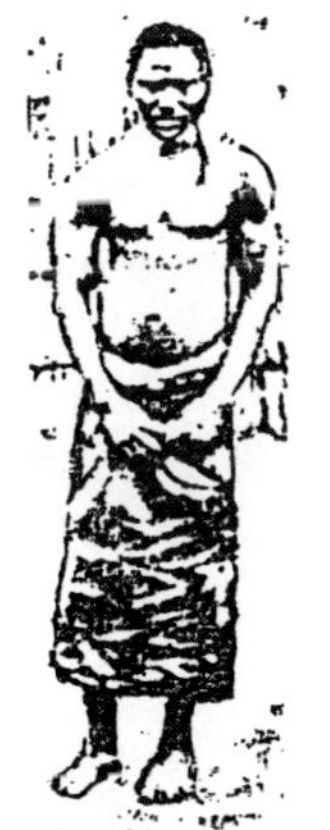

Mawalera Tembo

As William Koyi lay dying at Njuyu in June 1886, news came that the Ngoni Indaba had approved of Christian schools for their children. Sixty children arrived at the first school, and its success prompted Chief M'mbelwa to say: "you must not cultivate your garden merely in one place", other villages would be jealous without schools. Like Dr.Laws, Elmslie understood that a simple education is the essential precursor of all other progress.

Miss Janet Grant sailed out from Scotland to marry Walter Elmslie at the Blantyre Mission in September 1886. He bravely brought her, as the only Azungu woman around, to his house at Njuyu. Chief M'mbelwa greeted him - "yesterday you were a boy, today you are a man and can speak." The married state enhanced Dr.Elmslie's reputation among the Ngoni. "Matrimony has been more helpful to my work than celibacy".

Elmslie felt he was happier with one Christian wife than the polygamists around him! He wrote: "the multitude of his wives do not bring a man happiness; the wordy warfare is often sharp and long." A man had five wives and they were quarrelling; the husband said 'I love you all my wives' but they replied: 'why did you take us from our father's house seeing you only loved one of us?'

"Chief M'mbelwa asked me for a lock-up box to prevent his 30 wives stealing from him." "A husband might come home and find a crowd about his door and learn that one wife had taken muave, poison cup. He would bring her to me for an emetic, sometimes the patient died at my dispensary door."

"The young chief at Hora has quickly learned all the vices: beer drinking, hemp smoking, numerous wives, begging."

"The powerful men capture slave wives, the rich men buy all the marriageable girls of the tribe; often a grey-haired old man, with a dozen wives already, is bidding for the young girls of the tribe. Disparity of age, emotions, and associations, makes such unions very unhappy, and nowhere do quarrels and witchcraft practices foment more surely than in a polygamous household."

Mrs.Elmslie started sewing classes for the schoolgirls, but within a few months she became very ill with malaria - "I might mention that my wife being almost dead, was saved by being fed with raw beef juice. The Ngoni knew she was apparently dying and were tenderly sympathetic. When I had a bullock killed, they knew it was for her. The rumour went round that despite all my preaching, I did exactly as they did, and sacrificed a beast to my ancestral spirits!"

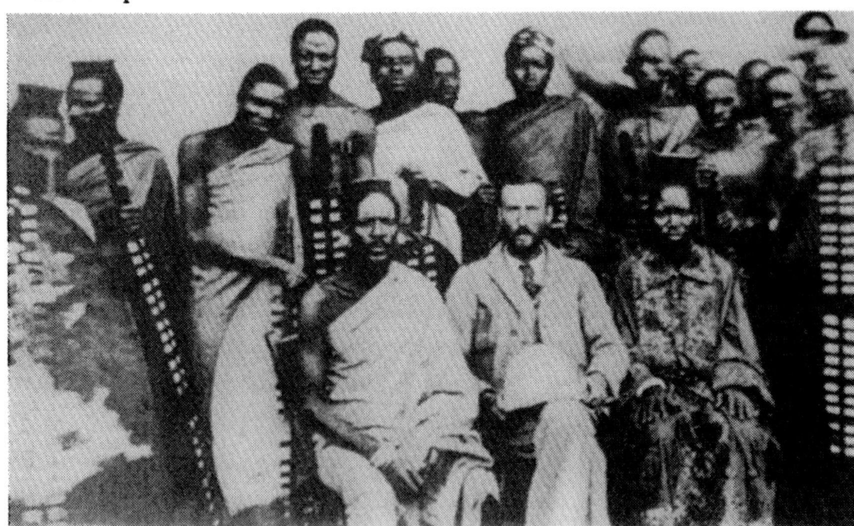

Dr. Elmslie and Chiefs

In July 1887, more trouble came. The Lakeshore Tonga around Bandawe had attacked the Ngoni, and were refusing to return captured women and children. Great Ngoni preparations were made for battle at Njuyu. "At this time we suffered from a severe family affliction and my wife was in bed. Around us were the Ngoni in a very unsettled state, engaging in war dances every day. Below our house, near the river, were encamped the armies of Chief Mtwalo and Chief Mabulabo, ready for war."

Dr.Elmslie sent secret messengers by night over the Viphya Mountains to Dr.Laws at Bandawe. The Laws were preparing to escape across the Lake if necessary. Elmslie wrote that the war spirit was rising, the Impis (regiments) were dancing and ready to march, and that Mrs.Elmslie was very ill, too ill to travel to Bandawe. Laws replied "your safety and success lies in delay and in holding on quietly if possible." He advised Elmslie to send all his surgical instruments and microscope to Bandawe, which he did. The parcels were carried secretly over the mountains by Tonga messengers. Dr.Elmslie then packed all his books in boxes and decided to bury them underground at Njuyu Village, along with the medicines in his well stocked dispensary: "It was the height of the dry season and the ground was as hard as a stone. I went out for several nights at one o'clock, and with an augur bored out the ground under cover of darkness, and scooped the earth out with my hands. I dared not use any tool lest the sound should attract attention...my wife was lying weak and helpless in bed, no doubt greatly hindered in her convalescence by the anxieties of the time. For several hours every night I dug up the earth and made pits in which to bury the medicines, anon running in to pass a few moments with my wife in her weakness. I sent a plan of the spots where things were hidden to Bandawe."

The Ngoni warriors were clamouring for Dr.Laws, and at last he came, sick with fever, to the Great Indaba with Chief M'mbelwa at Njuyu, on October 27th 1887. This meeting began at 8 a.m. and Dr.Laws had to sit in the hot tropical sun in the Kraal for eight hours. The Ngoni problems were resolved when the powerful Chief Mtwalo asked for a Christian doctor at Ekwendeni. The Ngoni could not approve of all the help being given to the Tonga people. The real reason why war was prevented though was because everybody respected Dr.Laws.

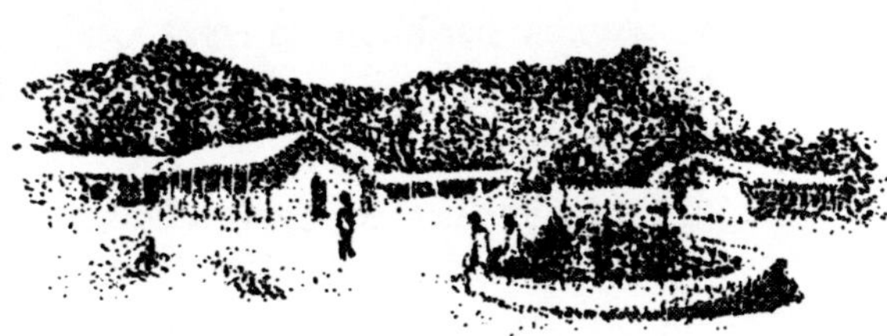

Njuyu today. Dr.Elmslie's house was by the circular flower bed in the foreground

Elmslie wrote "living as I did near Chief M'mbelwa for six years before he died, I know that he stopped the Ngoni from attacking the Tonga only because of his regard and affection for Dr.Laws, and not because of his belief in God." However, Walter Elmslie too had won the trust of the Ngoni. He had been the first doctor to visit Chief Mtwalo, and now..."we received a hearty welcome at Ekwendeni. When Mtwalo's son who had been sick, was brought out and proudly shown to be in good health through the white man's medicine, it was evident that the effects of medical work were wider than the boy's recovery." "Some days were spent at Chief Mtwalo's Village (Ekwendeni), and a frank invitation to remain was addressed to us. They had heard of the medical work and they wanted a medical man...they were not sure if their children should be taught...they offered a site for our house and garden, and requested us to come and build." Two more years of work at Njuyu came first, and then in 1890 the Mission extended its work in Ngoniland. Five schools were opened, dispensaries were built, and Dr.George Steele came to work in Chief Mzukuzuku's* district at Hora.

Walter Elmslie was a close friend of his fellow Aberdonian, Robert Laws. In 1890, he hurried over the Viphya Mountains, through thunderstorms and torrential rains which flooded the rivers, to a very sick Dr.Laws at Bandawe. He was forced to sit all night under bushes for shelter, with wild animals prowling round.

Dr.Elmslie's strict manner and direct honesty was valued by the Ngoni, but upset some Europeans. Andrew Murray of Mvera wrote of "Elmslie, in his usual sharp way...." and noted that "a good deal of grace was needed to get on with him, and corresponding with him was not very profitable to the spiritual life." Yet a convivial picture was depicted of him by his fellow missionaries. The guest house at Bandawe was destroyed by lightening at Christmas in 1892. So Walter and Janet Elmslie took into their house many outcasts who greatly enjoyed their Christmas dinner. Similar pleasure was recorded when the Elmslie party came on ulendo to Njuyu Village in 1893 ..."we enjoyed their visit very much." Mrs.Elmslie nursed staff who were sick, whilst her husband went to see Chief Mzukuzuku with Dr.Steele, to negotiate a site for a new mission at Hora. This Chief brought one of his wives to call on her.

In 1894, Elmslie accompanied Dr.Laws on the expedition to look for the final site for Livingstonia at Kondowe. As they camped by the Lake, three lions appeared and tore at their tent in the night. Yuria Chirwa raised the alarm, and helped fend off these animals.

* Illus. inside back cover

Dr.Elmslie usually took charge of Livingstonia when Dr.Laws went on leave, as in 1901 when a serious smallpox epidemic occurred at Kondowe: "segregation camps were promptly formed by Dr.Elmslie and grass huts erected for the treatment of patients. Only one death occurred."

In 1902, Ekwendeni Mission reported: "Dr.Elmslie's house is now finished and commands a magnificent view of Ngoniland. It can be seen 12 miles away."

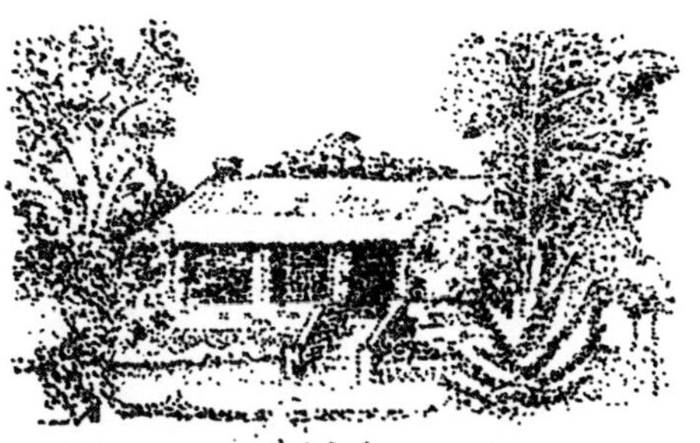

Dr.Elmslie's house.

Quietly medical work expanded amongst the Ngoni. In 1903, Hora station reported 3,663 patients, including many serious cases "which could not be dealt with for lack of a hospital. As bricks have been made by the people for a cottage hospital, it is hoped we will be able to erect it, by the free labour of the people." Other dispensary and hospital buildings were similarly erected in Ngoniland.

In 1911, Dr.Elmslie was given a motor-bike, and could travel easily on the 180 miles of road which had just been made in the area. The technology of the twentieth century was arriving. The first ringed bird seen in Nyasaland was sighted in April 1913 by Walter Elmslie, in a garden near Kacheche. It was a crane, with the mark "Ormuth Koypout Budapest Hungaria 4811". He was also a scholar. He was the first person to put the Tumbuka language in writing, and he translated the Gospels into Tumbuka.

He also wrote books about "The Wild Angoni", in which he depicts vividly both the problems and the loveliness of the old Ngoni way of life .... "In the sunset comes the folding of the cattle. The herd boys have reeds which they blow to make musical sounds, different herds having reeds of different pitches. They all sound together to produce simple sweet music. The nsima is cooked in one huge pot, and the men and women eat it separately. Then, if it is dry and the moon is up, the youths and maidens go to the Cattle Kraal to dance. The song is the principal thing, telling the story of their history, and the dance rhythms accompany it. The men, with their dancing sticks held up in their hands, form one line, and the women another. They strike the ground with their feet, while the sticks are waved overhead, and the bodies undulate. The notes rise and fall in the evening stillness."

A century later, the grandsons of the first Ngoni Christians still remember Dr.Elmslie: "he favoured us all, he was very strict but he loved and cared for us."

12   ACID FAST BACILLI

The bacteria that cause tuberculosis and leprosy have many similarities. They are very slow growing, and both have an outer coat that prevents the dye used to stain them for examination under the microscope from being washed away by acids (acid fast). The diseases they cause are both chronic, and the living conditions and immunity of the patient play an important part. When the incidence of the disease is studied today, the similarities end. Tuberculosis in Africa is taking on epidemic proportions, whereas leprosy is declining in Malaŵi.

TUBERCULOSIS (TB)

"The weariness, the fever, and the fret, here where men sit and hear each other groan." (John Keats who trained as a doctor and died of TB in 1821).

"Today I found one of my patients dead in the dispensary lying curled up in his blanket as he always used to lie. He died of consumption and, poor chap, he was an awful skeleton." (Wordsworth Poole 1895 at Zomba)

Robert Koch, who in 1882 identified the TB bacillus, said that in Germany then 1 in 7 deaths were caused by tuberculosis. The early missionaries, including Livingstone, were therefore pleased to find how rare it was in Central Africa.

Dr.Howard of Likoma Island wrote in 1910 "TB was rare 10 years ago, only seen along the slave and trade routes, and in certain families." It was already increasing even then, probably from South Africa, and in the same year there were 10 proved cases among 97 returning miners. The Annual Government Health Report noted "legislation will be necessary to prevent such an infection from being introduced among a population which to a marked extent must be more or less non-immune." The number of cases reported increased steadily."At one time we had 2 cases of pulmonary phthisis in our wards and we have heard of others. If cases of this kind become numerous they will require accommodation separate from other patients in the interest of all concerned."(Livingstonia 1915)

It is interesting that the first named death from TB in the country was of Shadrach Nguna in 1877 at Cape Maclear. He was one of the African missionaries from Lovedale in South Africa working with Dr.Laws.

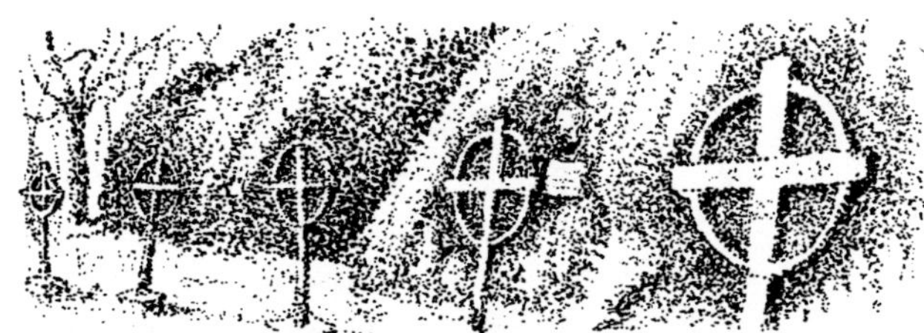

ιn Europe at this time, there was a fall in the death rate from TB due to improved housing, nutrition, and Public Health legislation. This was long before any useful drugs were available. Little of a similar nature could be done in Nyasaland then, and the patients were usually sent home, thereby infecting others. The outlook was poor, and most patients would have died.

Penicillin was not effective in tuberculosis, but hope for sufferers came in the 1950s. Dr.Waksman, a soil bacteriologist working in the U.S.A. was investigating why TB bacilli did not survive in the soil. He found that a soil fungus produced a substance he called streptomycin that killed them. This was found to be useful first in animals and then in humans with TB, although the bacteria tended to become resistant. Later other chemicals were used in combination with streptomycin to prevent this resistance developing.

The problem in Nyasaland worsened. By 1948 "the real incidence of TB is unknown; it is on the increase, and in the past 20 years a threefold rise has occurred in notifications." In Zomba Hospital there were no beds set aside for TB patients in 1951. Dr.Goodall was working there and took an interest in diagnosing and treating TB patients with new drugs. He was allowed to house the patients on the khonde (up to 70 at a time). 193 TB patients were admitted between 1951-3. They were mostly aged 20-30 years, and stayed for 3 months. Streptomycin (by injection) was given although supplies were variable and inadequate. In 1955 there were 32.3 per 100,000 new cases per year.

Two years later a TB Specialist was appointed as well as a Radiologist. Relentlessly the numbers increased. By 1958 "TB is making such strides that it overshadows the other disease problems."(Government Health Report). By 1962 there were 800 hospital beds occupied by TB patients. Many would abscond during

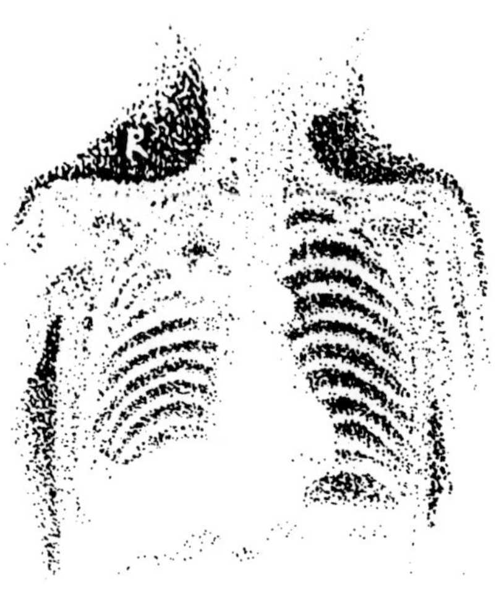

X-ray showing TB of R.lung.

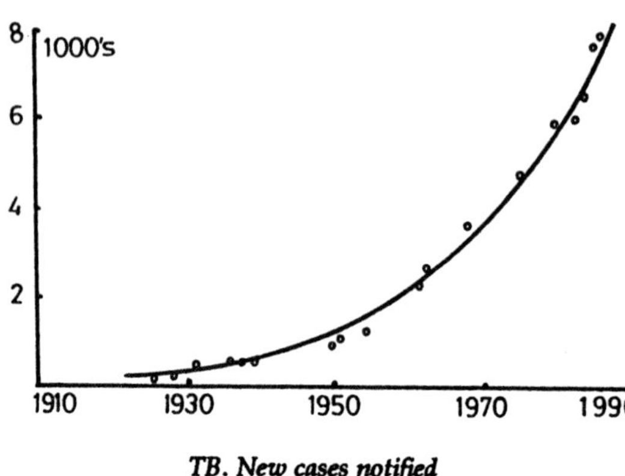

TB. New cases notified

the long course of treatment. A follow up study in 1969 of 1,708 confirmed patients showed 47% were responding to treatment, 30% were lost to follow up, and 22% died or remained sputum positive (due to a failure to take treatment or bacterial resistance). In this year the incidence in the Malaŵian population had risen to 38 per 100,000 and nearly 3,500 patients were admitted for treatment.

By 1982 the incidence had more than doubled: 80 new cases per year per 100,000 of the people. BCG was given to children but it was not clear whether this was beneficial. (BCG is a weakened strain of bacteria given to stimulate immunity).

TB is the 8th most common cause of death in Malaŵian hospitals, but many sufferers will die at home. There is an organized but overworked TB reporting and follow-up system, and treatment can be given on an outpatient basis. A powerful new, but expensive, antibiotic Rifampicin, which can be given by mouth is being used and this can shorten the treatment time. In 1988 over 8,000 new cases were reported as the numbers continue to increase. Many patients were HIV positive and may not respond well to treatment. The situation is similar to other African countries, and the epidemic continues.

LEPROSY

"Ten men were lepers which stood afar off' St. Luke 17,1

"I hope that the time will come - it may not be in our time, it could be in our children's children, when they will sit back and look at this day, and say, those people were far sighted, the last leprosy case has gone from Malaŵi." (Prime Minister Dr.H.K. Banda at the signing of the LEPRA agreement, 1965).

The last indigenous case of leprosy in Britain died in the Shetland Isles in 1798. The early missionaries were dismayed to see the ravages of the disease in Africa. "Endomoschule came up with his leprosy for a cure; his hands and his feet are swollen and so are his eyebrows and his nose. All his body is covered with it. He has two wives." (Livingstone at Magomero, 1862).

The leprosy of the Bible was probably often a mistranslation, but its dread association caused a change of name and 'Hansen's Disease' is often used. He was a doctor in Norway. Although Pasteur in 1866 in France had shown that spoiling and souring of milk and wine was due to bacteria, Hansen was the first to show a human disease was due to a bacteria when he described the leprosy bacillus in 1874. He also tried experimentally to infect himself with bacteria from one of his patients, luckily without success. He must have had a high degree of immunity, his wife had died some years previously of tuberculosis and he did not catch it. There is probably a degree of cross-immunity between the two diseases which have several points of similarity.

Blood tests in Malaŵi show that today most of the population over six years old have had contact with the leprosy bacillus, most develop a complete immunity, less than 2% develop the disease. Even within the disease itself, a degree of immunity gives the patient a certain type (called confusingly 'tuberculoid') with damage to nerves and few bacteria to be found in the tissues. When there is no immunity, the person develops lepromatous leprosy with the tissues swarming with bacteria, such as Endomoschule, described above.

Dr.Robert Howard on Likoma Island in 1910 under-estimated the incidence to be 1/1,000 of the population. He said the leper was not regarded as an outcast but had a separate shelter under the eaves of a house and ate his food separately. There was a belief at that time that a fish diet had something to do with the disease. 53 cases were observed in 1910 but only 4 came for treatment.

Various isolation areas were set up. One was on Lundu Island where the entire population were lepers.The UMCA missionaries came regularly on the **Chauncy Maples** to give treatment,and even in the First World War in 1914 the Germans on the nearby Tanganyikan coast supplied some food to this colony. "The lepers grow some food and they have cleared a good path around the island and keep it free from weeds." The apathy and tedium of their lives was hard to bear. By 1924 the UMCA missions were treating 332 cases with increasing doses of injections of moogrol. This was an extract of Chaulmoogrol oil, an ancient remedy from an Asian plant. Patients however did not persist with the treatment which was of questionable value.

In 1927, at Zomba, a leprosy conference was held and a lantern lecture given that was open to the public. In the same year supplies of Hydnocarpus oil from Calcutta arrived "probably better than Chaulmoogrol". 220 patients were treated with 5,489 injections. The oil was like golden syrup and in the cool weather had to be warmed before it could be injected. "The patients bore the insertions of the large needle with considerable fortitude, only a wry face indicated pain. All were busy massaging the skin with a bloodstained grey swab; some rubbed each other when the site was inaccessible." "People accepted the diagnosis philosophically, I never had to resort to the use of any euphemism or beat about the bush. I merely said 'nkate'(leprosy).'Chabwino!'(Good) was the usual reply, and with no hut tax to pay some thought it a fairly good exchange. I have never heard one rave or curse." (Malosa nurse 1940's).*

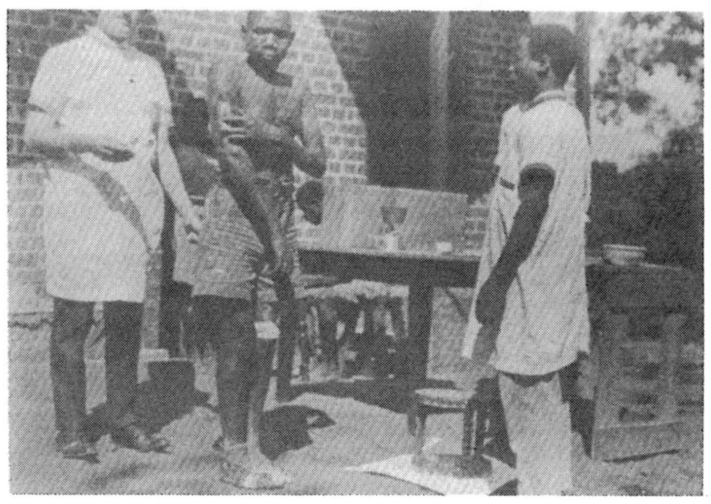

Oil injections, Malamulo 1930

LEPROSY CENTRES IN THE 1930's

UMCA	Likoma, Malindi, Likwenu
CCAP	Bandawe, Livingstonia,
	Domasi, Loudon, Nkhoma (DRC)
SDA	Malamulo (230 patients), Mwami
CATHOLIC	Mua, Utale

In 1935 one European under treatment had been pronounced free of the disease.

Dr.Muir of the British Empire Leprosy Relief Association did a survey in 1939 and visited all the centres."It is the first visit we have ever had from a specialist, and he taught us much in the days he spent with us." There were 755 inmates (twice as many men as women) and 436 outpatients. He recommended centralisation of services and employment of more full time

* *Illus. inside back cover.*

health workers. Ten years later there were 942 inpatients and 436 outpatients, and in 1951 sulphones were used for the first time. This was a great advance in treatment and could be given by mouth. "A spirit of hope has replaced the previous gloom and apathy among the patients."

The incidence of cases continued to increase however. In 1953 it was estimated at 1·4%. A Mulanje survey in 1955 showed that 1·6% of the population had leprosy (17% lepromatous). In 1952 the Brown Memorial Fund for Leprosy was bequeathed in memory of the founder of the tea industry (£232,000).

In 1965 the British Leprosy Relief Association (LEPRA) initiated a pilot control project based on treatment at home of patients in the early stages of the disease. 4,000 patients were under active treatment by 1966. By the end of 1970, 11,000 had been registered, and 220 discharged cured. Work then expanded from Blantyre to the whole of Malaŵi.

In 1983 a powerful new drug Rifampicin was added to the treatment schedules with very impressive results, cases per 100,000 falling from 38.3 in 1978 to 13.7 in 1987. By 1981, the number of patients cured equalled the number of new cases (2,000). In 1988 there were less than 1,000 new cases reported for the first time since adequate records were kept.

Because of its high reputation in the leprosy field throughout the world, Malaŵi was chosen in 1986 for a major trial of vaccine in the Karonga area. The vaccine is produced in an armadillo, one of the very few animals in which the leprosy bacillus will multiply apart from man. Over the next decade it should become clear whether this will be the means of eliminating the disease.

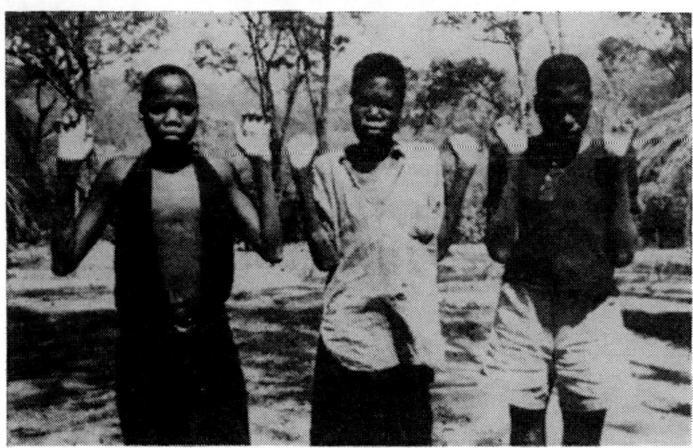

1930 Leprosy patients.

Since 1973 the Seventh Day Adventists at Malamulo Hospital, Makwasa, have organized the control centre for the Lower Shire Valley. In the 1930s they had the largest leprosarium in the country.

SEVENTH DAY ADVENTISTS

The first clinic was opened at Makwasa, near Thyolo, by Nurse Irene Fourie in 1915. Dr.Carl Birkenstock arrived from South Africa in 1925 and within a few years began leprosy work. A small ward for lepers eventually grew into a large unit. In 1973, Malamulo Hospital became the Leprosy Control Centre for the Lower Shire Valley, in addition to general hospital work. In 1935, a Medical Assistants' Training School was started at Makwasa, and has trained students to a consistently high standard. Attractive buildings constructed during the past decade, make this hospital one of the most up-to-date in Malaŵi. The hospital is financially supported by the Adventist Church of the U.S.A., and it is mainly staffed by American doctors and specialists. Malamulo Hospital in Blantyre is also a busy private hospital, and the Adventists also operate several rural health centres.

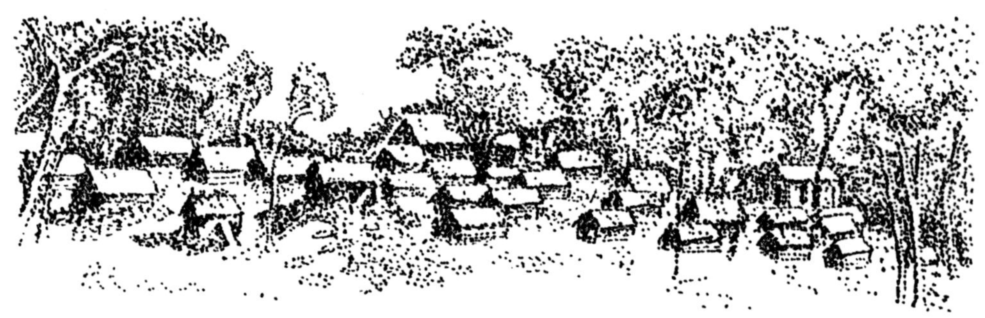

Leper Colony, Malamulo 1930.

On October 23rd 1876, a party of Church of Scotland missionaries pitched their tents under a fig tree near Ndirande Mountain. The site had been selected by Henry Henderson because it was away from the main slave trade route to Mulanje and Quelimane. The missionaries named this place Blantyre after David Livingstone's native town in Scotland. This was the romantic origin of the modern city of Blantyre.

From the beginning, this was a medical mission, staffed by a continuous succession of dedicated doctors. Dr.Macklin was the first, and "Mr.Henderson and Dr.Macklin have lived in a round hut 15 foot in diameter, crowded with goods, for six months" wrote James Stewart in 1877.

The first decade was filled with problems from run-away slaves, and tribal raids. In October 1884 the Ngoni raided the Shire Highlands, and the Mission became a sanctuary for hundreds of fleeing Africans. Consul Foot arrived to try to maintain law and order. By 1891,"a few Ngoni are beginning to venture across now with their sheep and goats for sale among the people...a hush comes over a group as even a single member of that tribe passes by."

The first surgical operation was done by Dr.Laws (seconded from Cape Maclear) on the manse dining room table there in 1880. In 1887, Dr.John Bowie gave up a lucrative London practice to come to Blantyre. He built the first hospital of grass and clay which was locally known as St.Bartholemew's, after his London hospital. Unfortunately the first patient admitted, died there. So great was the fear of witchcraft, that no one else would enter. Dr.and Mrs.Bowie had to take patients into their own house instead.

The pioneering difficulties were considerable:" Makata, the man who had his arm removed, deserves honourable mention....he knew nothing of the virtues of chloroform, and repeated 'the people of my village say: No, do not have it off; it will be very sore; but they are women'. His attitude was an act of courage, a jump into the profundity of the unknown."(Blantyre Report 1890)

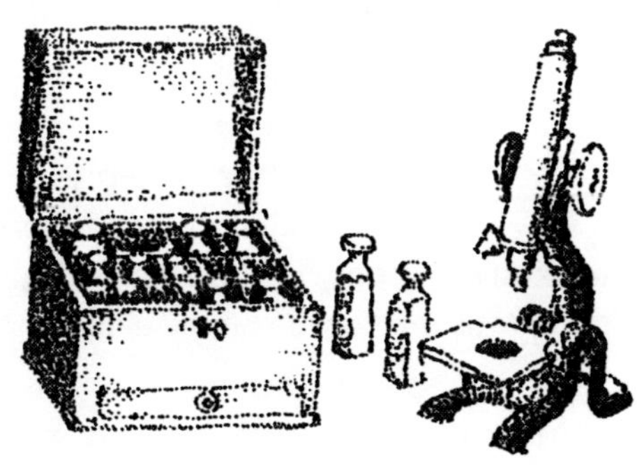

Medicine chest and microscope used in Blantyre Mission c.1900.Blantyre Museum.

Then a diphtheria tragedy occurred: "A baby son (8 months) of Henry Henderson, who had married a sister of Dr.Bowie, was attacked with diphtheria, and died. In a few days the mother followed. In a vain attempt to save the child's life, Bowie sucked the tube inserted after a tracheostomy operation, and caught the infection. He made all preparations for a similar operation on himself, for he was a skilled surgeon. He summoned a relative, Dr.Affleck Scott, from Mulanje. The latter, to cross the Thuchila River, swollen by torrential rains, made a bridge of bamboo from bough to bough of trees on either side. But all in vain! Bowie died, and was buried beside his sister; three deaths within 9 days in January 1891." Henry Henderson, a broken man, left to take Mrs.Bowie back to Britain, but on reaching Quelimane, at the mouth of the Zambesi River, they were stricken with fever, and both died there, brother in law and sister in law.

Bravely the medical missionaries continued their work. Dr.Affleck Scott (1862-95)* worked at Domasi Mission, Mulanje Mission, and finally at Blantyre. "It was quite common to see him on a shake down and an African patient in his best bed." He walked to surrounding villages and never spared himself. He was beloved by all races and had over 60 patients a day. At Blantyre, he helped his brother Clement mould the bricks for St. Michael's Cathedral.

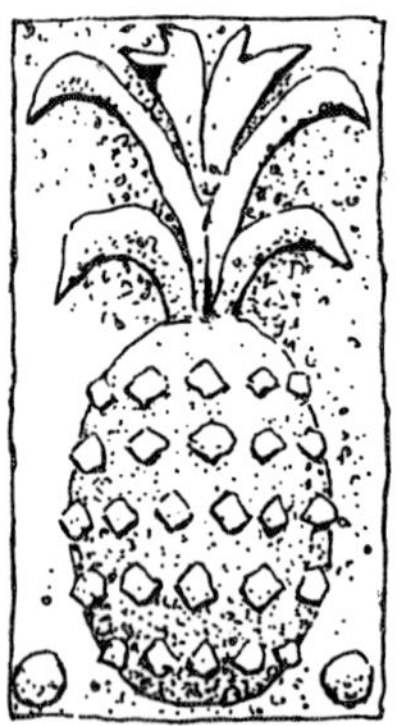

Intricate brick moulds were made by Affleck, including the pineapple and oak leaf bricks which can be seen in the Cathedral today. In 1895, he walked to Domasi to join Captain Manning's military expedition against Chief Kawinga's slave fort in the Chikala Hills.

With the first Government in 1891, more peaceful progress was possible. "The heliograph is now working between the Zomba Residency and Mulanje Mission. They are sending almost daily messages. The smoke prevents communication at midday, but in the early morning they are generally able to work. They are using only 5 inch glasses." Also in 1893, the road from Blantyre to Zomba was measured and milestones erected.

Blantyre Mission was the first stepping stone for many pioneers to British Central Africa. Arthur Fraser Sim described his visit in 1894, after a hazardous journey up from Quelimane: "Imagine my feelings when I found a group gathered around a blazing fire in a brick house with a real chimney, a long table laid out with a clean cloth. After falling upon our host's wardrobe, I soon set to work upon his larder. Blantyre is famous for its good fellowship and civilization."

Illus. inside front cover

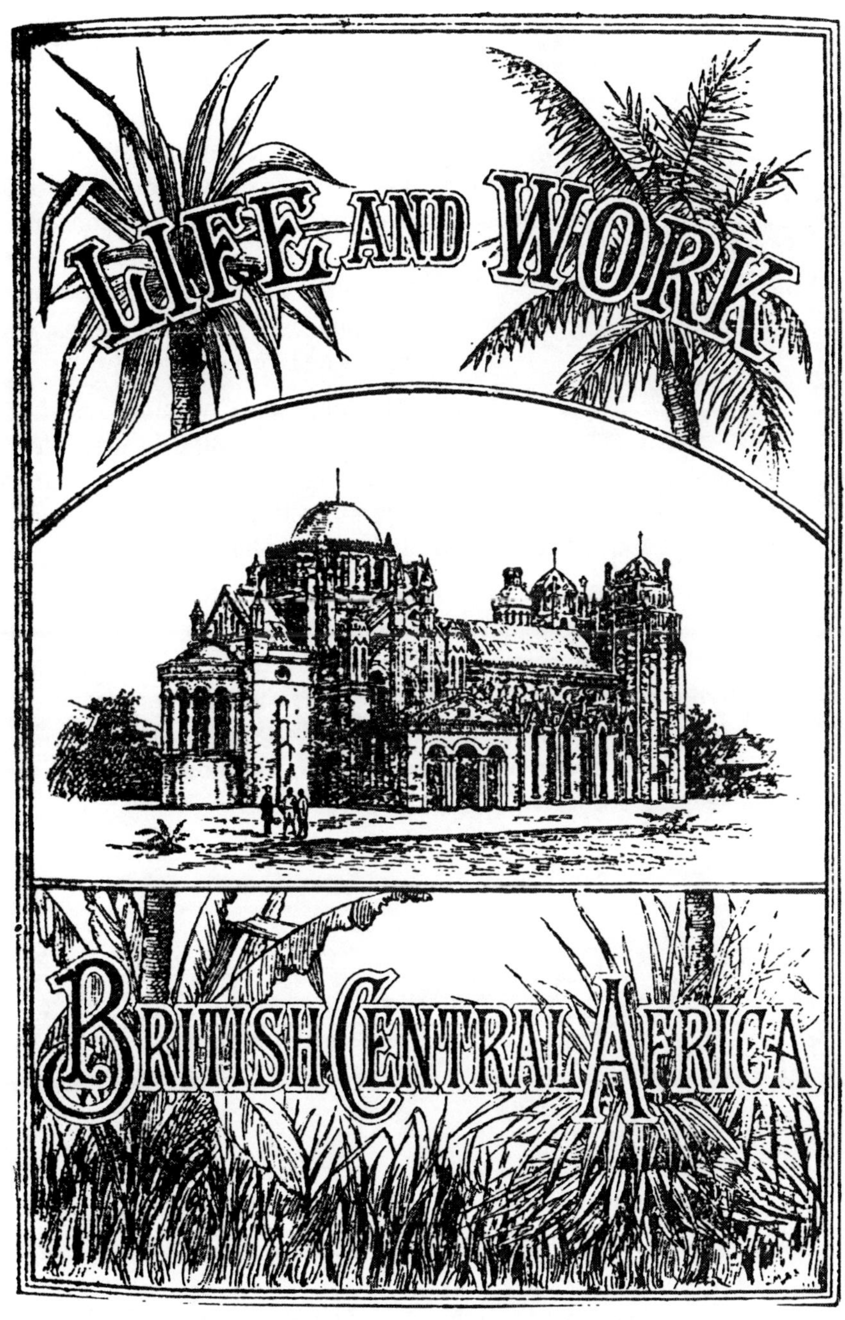

St. Michael's Church on Mission magazine cover.

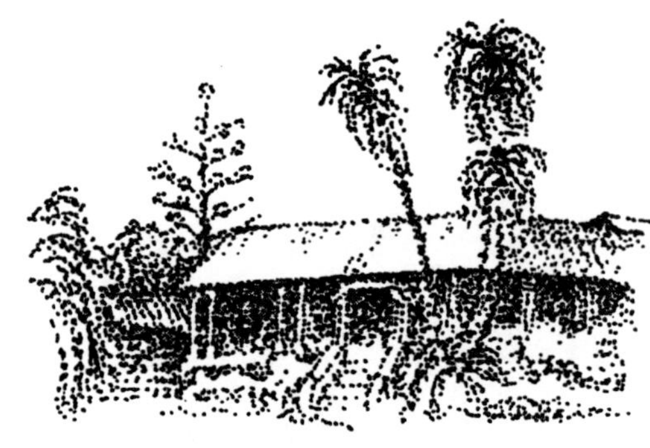

Blantyre Mission Hospital, now a school.

There was now an urgent need for a hospital. In 1894 Blantyre reported many gunshot wounds and animal injuries: "a man walked from the Upper Shire (30 miles) with his upper arm terribly mauled by a crocodile. At first he would not consent to amputation, but his pulse was rising, so we cut as low as possible." Blantyre Mission then had two rooms, each with a bed for a patient.

The first proper hospital was built in Blantyre Mission in 1896, with a male ward and an operating theatre, followed later by a female ward. Miss Farquar arrived from Edinburgh to start nursing, and Dr.MacVicar started to teach Hospital Assistants. Blantyre Mission's pioneering contribution to African medical education was very fine (see chapter on Training).

At Domasi Mission, plagues of locusts, lions, and leopards, all caused severe problems in 1896: "every man, woman, and child were in the gardens waving bits of cloth tied to bamboos, beating empty tins and anything else, to drive off the locusts". "At Chikala, a lion carried off one of Mposa's wives from her hut door, parts of her body were found in the Bush, we have great difficulty keeping our fowls."

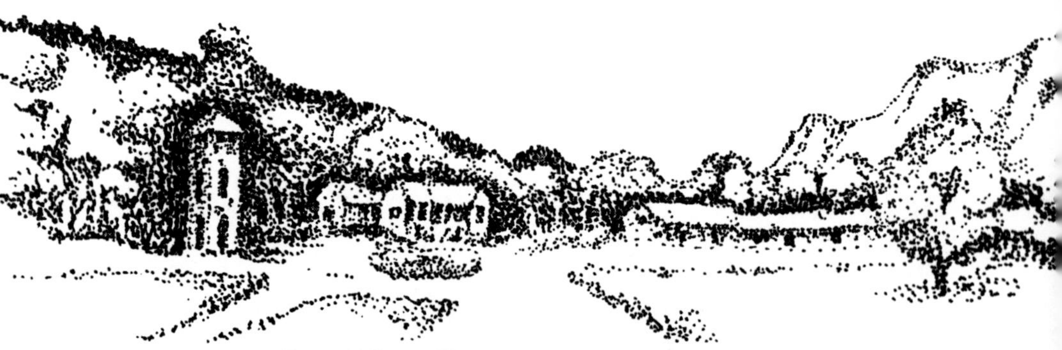

Domasi Mission Hospital on left to the right of the Bell Tower..

In the beautiful Domasi Valley of the Zomba Massif, the doctor saw patients on the verandah of his house, and did operations in his dining room. The local people by their own free labour made bricks, and then built Domasi Mission Hospital, in 1903.

By 1902, Blantyre Hospital boasted four buildings of burnt brick roofed with corrugated iron. Then a medical improvement came with cement floors instead of mud ones. The fame of these floors spread across Nyasaland, and Reuben, the Medical Dresser from Embangweni came down to see them, and returned to make them at Loudon Hospital. The Livingstone Mission Hospital at Zomba noted "cement floors are unknown here, and greatly desired, especially in the operating room. There is no lack of patients here."

In June 1904, there was a big day in the Blantyre Mission when 62 iron hospital beds arrived from Scotland: "The beds at last! The number of patients we admit however bears no relation to the number of beds, we had to put 39 patients into 28 beds in the male ward the night they arrived."

The Scottish Mission Hospitals at Blantyre, Mulanje, Zomba, and Domasi, made a great contribution to health services and to medical education in the South for half a century. Blantyre Mission Hospital was transferred into the new Queen Elizabeth Hospital when it opened in 1958. Mulanje Mission Hospital continues today with an emphasis on maternity work.

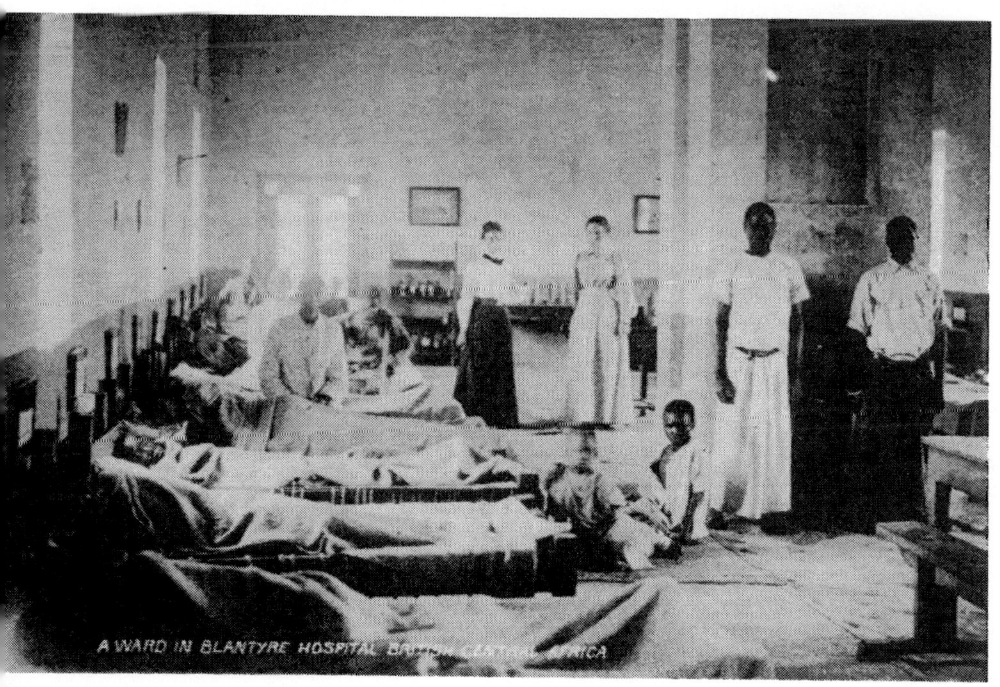

Blantyre Hospital Ward c.1900.

BLANTYRE EUROPEAN HOSPITAL

On August 2nd 1895 a public meeting was held in Blantyre Court House, with John Buchanan in the chair, to discuss the proposal "Blantyre Mission have advised an independent scheme for a public hospital, as they are no longer able to provide hospital and public medical services." The white population of the Shire Highlands was increasing fast and was about 300.

The motion was passed with Major Forbes' support, £300 was raised there and then, and a committee established to construct it. The first hospital was opened before a large crowd on a ridge about three quarters of a mile from Blantyre Boma, overlooking the Chikwawa road, (above present day Jubilee Park),on May 3rd 1897. It was Queen Victoria's Diamond Jubilee Year. It contained four wards named Fotheringham, Buchanan, Scott, and Jubilee all with a good view. "The patients as they toilingly reach convalescence can enjoy the cricket matches which they overlook; and they will be by far the best people to consult for racing tips, seeing the race course lies beneath them, and the morning practice of the horses is in full view." (Scott) The first patient was a Mr.Runciman who had broken his leg at Thyolo.

In 1900 the Protectorate Administration took it over as a government hospital. As Blantyre grew, a new hospital was opened across the road in what is the present Health Office buildings in Victoria Avenue. This was the hospital for Europeans for half a century, until it was also transferred to the Queen Elizabeth Hospital for all races in 1958.

1950 saw the foundation of Newlands retirement homes for expatriates in Limbe, still well supported today.

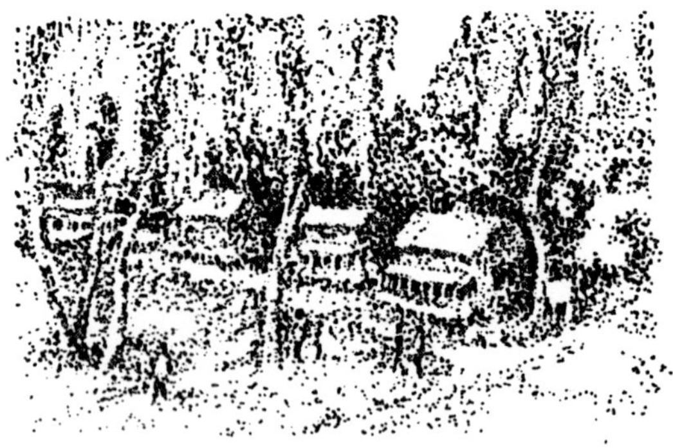

Old European Hospital Blantyre dwarfed by Eucalyptus trees.

14 DR. WORDSWORTH POOLE (served 1895-97)

"A charming and competent man, he possessed a magnetic personality that no one could resist" (R.Maugham 1895)

After a medical education at Cambridge (a First in Pathology) and Guy's Hospital, Dr.Poole arrived at Zomba in June 1895 as the British Central Africa government medical officer. Zomba was then a town with 6 brick houses. He was plunged immediately into the medical and surgical problems of patients without hospitals, and the adventurous military expeditions against the slave traders. His first task was to make a wooden leg for an African whose leg had been bitten off by a crocodile. Within a few weeks he built the first

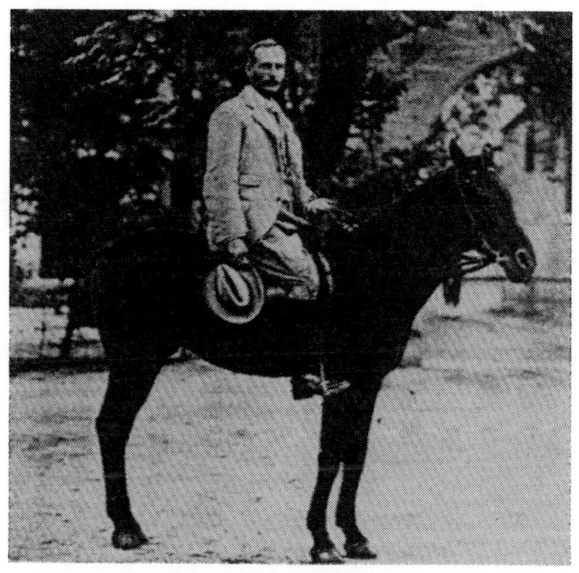

Dr Wordsworth Poole.

mud dispensary in Zomba. He wrote "this man was put in my dispensary and there he lay. One has to do everything oneself; all the nursing, feeding, preparing food, sitting up at night. My first three operations were successful, so a reputation soon gets around of the Mzungu (white man) who cuts away bits of the body without pain."

Then "Dr.Poole and the B.C.A. Administration are to be congratulated on having opened the first African hospital (as far as we know worthy of the name) in British Central Africa. The new hospital in Zomba is a neat, unassuming looking building, containing two large wards and an operating room. There are comfortable looking fireplaces neatly built of burnt brick, in all the rooms." (Domasi Mission Report 1895)

Dr. Poole loved the trekking life of Africa."Stewart and I walked to Liwonde, camping out for four nights.This roving life is very nice, pitching camp where there is water.You come in from a long day's march tired, covered with dust, hungry, have a bath, get into clean clothes, then the fires are lit all

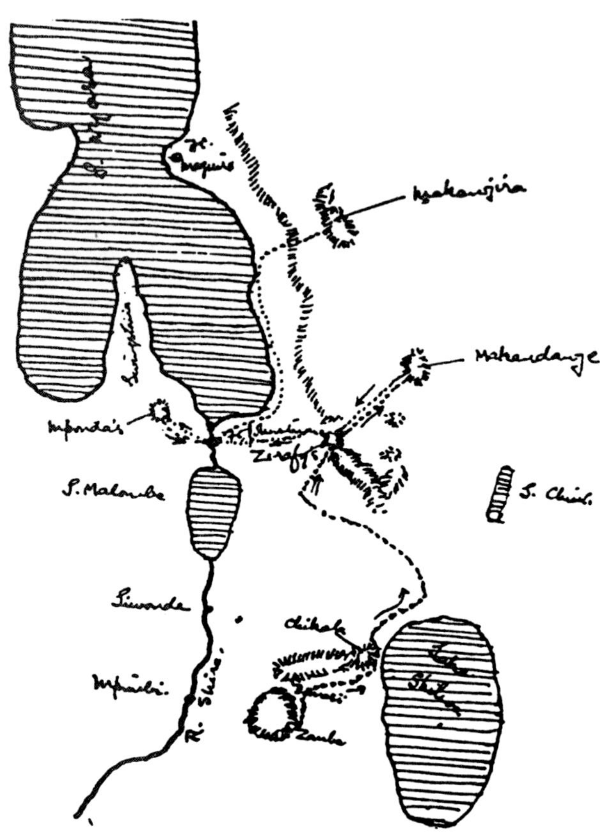

Campaign Map from a letter to his mother.

among the trees, the Africans sit around cooking, talking, and singing. The Tonga are always singing, today the song was: 'War, jolly fine war, and another wife for me."

He was soon summoned to accompany military expeditions against the slavers, under the command of Major C.A.Edwards, who had brought a Company of 100 Sikhs from India to serve beside 300 local Africans. The first encounter was with Chief Chawinga in the Chikala Hills: "A Makua has shot himself through the foot and made a fearful hole...I did not see him until four days afterwards, and the wound was in an awful state of putrefaction."

In August 1895 he joined the final campaign against Chiefs Zirafi(Jalasi) and Makanjila on the south east side of Lake Nyasa. "Dr.Rendell is coming to look after the Zomba hystericals while I am away, now I am looking at guns, revolvers, ammunition, kit..."

"I and my hospital carriers started a long trail up the steep ascent to the hills where Zirafi's Village stood. Zirafi's men stood tight in this impregnable fortress, dancing, and jeering at us from the tops of the rocks. But they did not like our rifles, and fled. Their women were shouting (not very drawing room language), and beating drums." Zirafi fled to Mozambique, and a British fort was built in his village. Chief Makanjila was also routed, and then Chief Mponda came personally to surrender all his slaves. They had come from all parts of Africa, including the Congo. Major Edwards freed all these slaves immediately.

Then the party embarked on Lake Nyasa to go up to Karonga,"that great Lake, so full of romance, so mixed up with everything African: slaves, dhows, Arabs, Coast men, travellers, missionaries, enterprises, traders, deaths, and treachery."

On the voyage, they stopped at Likoma Island,"I got myself into ill odour with the matron, a snappy little creature named Miss Woodward. There were two new lady missionaries who had just come out and had been nothing but ill since arrival. At Likoma Major Edwards had blackwater fever, I nursed him night and day. I also opened two deep abscesses in Major Bradshaw's thigh, and he required constant care, for his chloroform vomiting was troublesome."

On December 1st they reached Karonga by boat, and began the famous assault on the Slave Trader Mlozi's stockade: "there was a terrible hubbub of cows, and Africans, and Arabs; up on the wall and in amongst the houses was the most dangerous time." About 700 Nkonde men joined in the final attack on the stockade, from which Mlozi seemed to have disappeared. Sergeant Bandawe, a Tonga, bravely remained behind in the stockade and heard Mlozi speaking underground. He descended to a dugout chamber, threw himself at Mlozi's bodyguard, seized his spear, attacked Mlozi, and captured him.

Dr.Poole wrote "I had a busy night of it, dressing wounds, amputations, and horrible wounds among Mlozi's men...one of my patients was Mlozi himself. He had got a piece of bone driven into his skull into the dura mater, was semi-conscious and had a very bad scalp wound. I removed pieces of the bone, and next day he was quite sensible, sensible enough to be told that an Nkonde Council had sentenced him to death. He never showed the slightest fear or regret, and took his hanging like a man." So ended the terrible Lake Nyasa slave trade.

Back in Zomba, there was intense interest in the prospect of a European lady arriving, and Wordsworth Poole wrote: "if she is a chronic invalid, she will add to my woes. I do not think I possess a good ladies' bedside manner." "One does not miss Englishwomen in the least, and really does not think of them at all. When a paper with photographs of women turns up, one feels it would be nice to see a pretty woman again, just for the sake of seeing something good to look upon!"

He built his house next to Consul Harry Johnston's house (who was himself a remarkable man). "My cupboards are made of boxes placed on top of each other. Most of my tables are made of boxes too. A bamboo stretches across

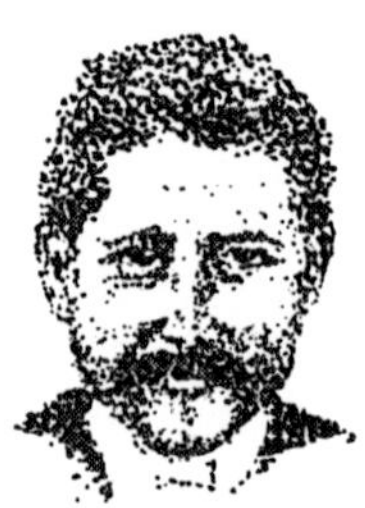

H.*Johnston*

the room, and from it hangs a large sheet of calico, which hides my bed and bath from the rest of the room."

He mentioned Harry Johnston as "very prim and proper: once my dispensary boy took brandy by mistake to some Hindi who were well instead of to some who were sick. Johnston sent a letter to say he did not wish people who were well to have brandy!"

As a pathologist, he was continually busy with "the excellent microscope Major Bradshaw gave me. I have made careful examinations of the blood and urine in cases of blackwater fever." He was continually absorbed with the African world around him. "The life is very fascinating, the camp fires, the odd journeys, the continual change of scene." And the local people found initiation into modern medicine a little alarming: "some quiver when they come, and one fled when I produced a stethoscope. One lady rushed away when I tried to examine her throat with a spatula."

"Once I had taken off a large fibrous growth from a patient, and another African said the white doctor was no good. An African medicine man would have given some medicine, and the growth would have disappeared." In a dysentery epidemic he noted "as soon as they are ill, they go away to the bush eating nothing because they feel no inclination, never for a moment thinking they must eat to live. Thus many have been carried to hospital in extremis, and died quickly."

Dr.Wordsworth Poole started Zomba Gymkhana Club, he rode a horse to Blantyre, he went on a leopard shoot, started a cricket club, and politicked for a library. In two years he contributed greatly to the country.

He described his evenings at home at Zomba: "It is a pretty sight from my verandah. The moon is up and the sky cloudless, and the mist over Shirwa seems to lead the sight into infinite space. Behind all is the imminent mass of Zomba Mountain. The groups of Africans round camp fires always fascinate me and make me wish I was African myself."

He wrote to his mother: "you would be quite surprised how very humdrum station life is out here. Yet alas for your hope for me as an English general practitioner. I feel I shall hanker for Africa.

> There was a young Cambridge M.B.
> Said I won't be a Cambridge G.P.
> But to Africa's shore
> I'll stick evermore
> And now he's a K.C.M.G." (honoured by a knighthood)

He enjoyed a trip on the Shire River; "our floating fiddle is going ahead tonight. The young moon has set, and we are zig-zagging part of the river. The stars give no light, but are reflected and enlarged lengthwise in the river water. To our right the Great Bear inverted, and then the Southern Cross. Fireflies flit about in pairs blinking their lights in the darkness.

Chiromo - A German trader, Hillier, has a nice bungalow and a piano. I had dinner on board, and then some music at Hillier's. At sundown we reached Hillier's camp about 6 miles upstream from Chiromo, and found they had already slain 3 waterbuck. The camp looked most picturesque. The green tent surrounded by reeds, in the distance the purple hills. Close by were several fires lighted by the boys, at which they were cooking their newly slain meat. We then had dinner in great style, put up the mosquito nets, had a smoke and went to bed."

"Put up for the night at an African Village. Bright moonlight. The villagers were sleeping on their mats in front of their thatched huts."

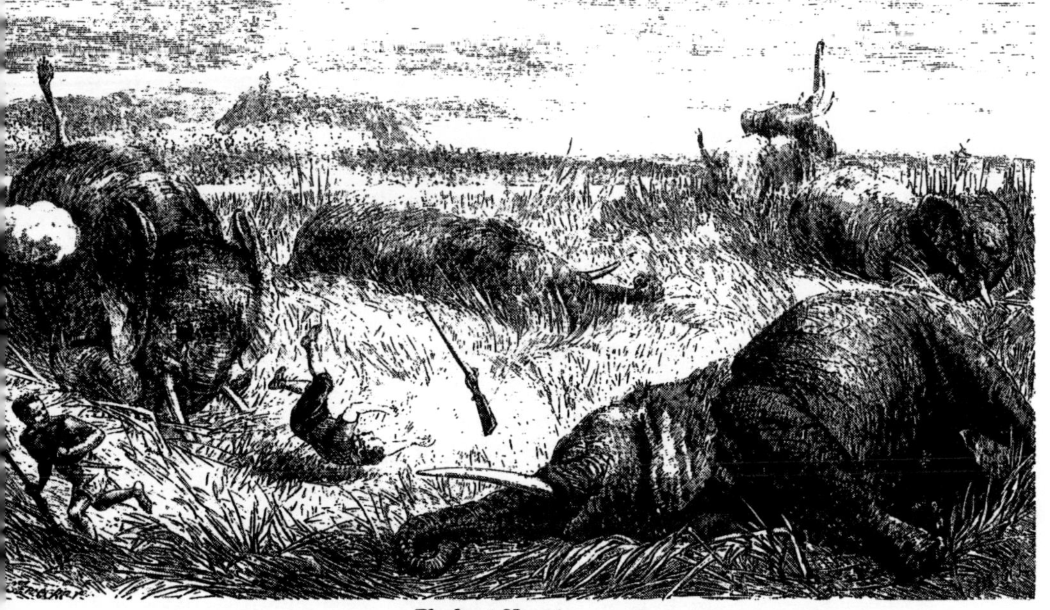

Elephant Haunts

He described going on ulendo to tend a man mauled by an elephant: "into the Utanga (basket) go pots, pans, spoons, cups, kettles, tin opener, rice tied up in a bag of calico, yarn, soap, cartridges, boots, bananas, pawpaws, and tobacco. A sack holds clothes, a waterproof sheet, blankets, and a dilapidated tent and poles. A sack of potatoes and maize meal, and a bed and chair, complete the outfit. I wear a sunhat, khaki knickerbockers, socks and boots. I can go at a fast pace. In a few days everything is filthily dirty and there has to be a general wash-up. The whole show looks like a rag shop."

"It's an odd sort of practice, where you travel 700 miles to see a patient and take a month over it. Johnstone did not make much improvement while I was at Likoma Island"...Johnstone was brought with Miss Rees, a British nurse to Zomba, after he had been mauled by an elephant near Likoma Islands, and badly injured.

"Miss Rees is staying up at the Residency, and Johnstone with me. He has had a very bad time of it. He had tetanus and erysipelas at Likoma and there are two great sloughs on his foot. The thigh has been broken in two places and the right shoulder bone is all smashed up. They have however both united, and in about two months time, he should be on his legs, and he will go home for good. Miss Rees is a good sort. She is very illiterate but a capital nurse and looked after Johnstone splendidly. The missionaries try to put a brake on her having a bit of enjoyment, much to her disgust. Poor Johnstone managed to get through after a very tight time."

After accompanying the expedition against Chief Gomani at Ntcheu, he wrote "by the by, I nearly got a new antelope called after me, the something; cornis Pooli, we found it in the Southern Ngoni Hills."

He tried drawing the African scene "at first I felt at sea sketching anything. Here everything is so extensive that it was difficult to fix attention on one aspect of the scene. The strong sunlight takes the colour out of everything; but when the sun is setting the country looks at its best."

Dr.Wordsworth Poole's happiness here was evident on his safari journeys. "At sundown we find a nice place to sleep in close to a river, have a meal and sit round the camp fire smoking. The boys sit talking until we turn in. Then all is quiet except for the call of the night jar and the occasional cry of a hyena. Sometimes a lion is heard, and the Africans are up the trees in a remarkably short time. Though there are a lot of lions about, one rarely sees them, and they are not often shot, for they are cunning beasts."

He enjoyed designing his home at Zomba: "you see the house will be fairly high. It will command a most exquisite view. There is water near it, which can be used for irrigation, so that it is possible to have a very good garden. As soon as it is built, I shall become partly farmer partly gardener, I hope to have cows. To be stranded without milk is an abomination, when one's drink is par excellence tea. I drink quarts of that. I have it four times a day."

Dr.Wordsworth Poole departed in June 1897. He joined Lugard's Ashanti Campaign in Ghana, and then went to Pekin as Legation doctor during the famous Siege of 1900. He died there of typhoid in 1902, aged 33 years. There is a memorial to him in the Legation Chapel at Pekin.

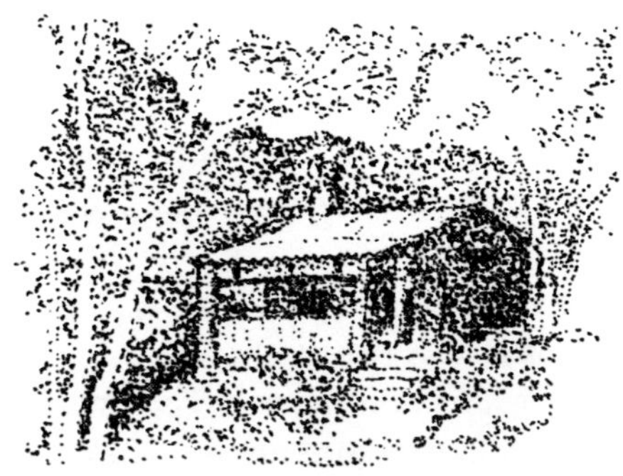

Dr Poole's House.

Malemia Top Hospital at Zomba is in the grounds chosen by Dr. Poole as his home in 1893. His little house overlooks the deep ravine of the Mponda stream, and is now a staff house.

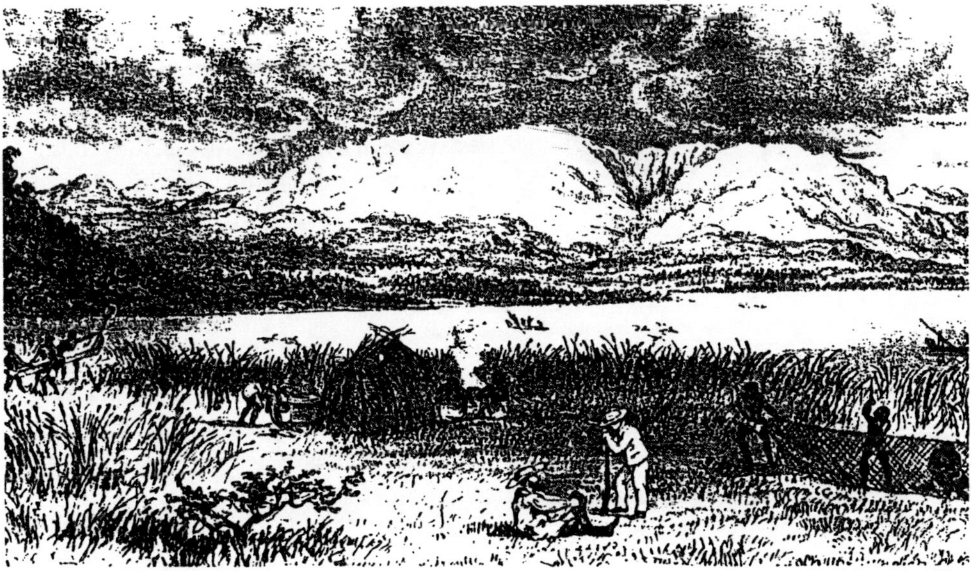

Fr. Schenck. 12 Rl. Exch., Edinr.

(C. Meller, Oct., 1861.

View of Zomba from Lake Chilwa from a drawing by Dr.Meller.

15 WORMS

Parasitic worms with their curious life cycles are a cause of much ill health in tropical countries including Malaŵi. Onchocerciasis occurs in a small pocket near Thyolo; it only causes minor skin lesions and not the devastating River Blindness seen in parts of Africa. Research is continuing in the country to find methods of control of the vector, the small black fly, simulum. Filariasis is seen in parts of Malaŵi causing fever and skin lesions. It is interesting historically because it was the first mosquito-transmitted disease described by Manson in China. This made him suggest a mosquito connection in malaria. Hydatid disease, due to a tape worm, although common on other East African countries, is very rare in Malaŵi.

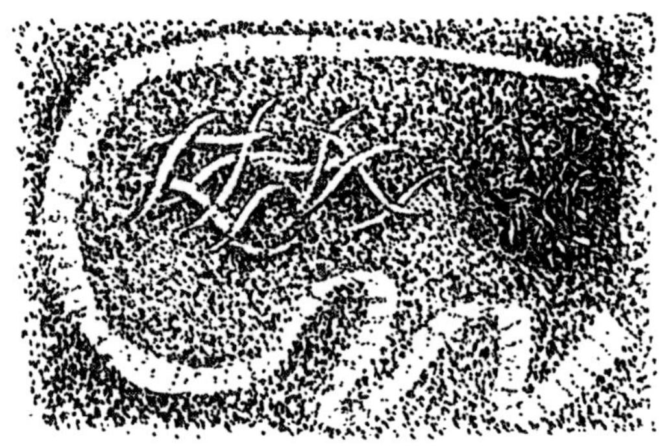

Three intestinal worms, roughly to scale. Tape, Round and Hookworm (one cm. long).

Tapeworms and roundworms are easily visible to the naked eye when passed, but usually do not cause serious symptoms. The smaller very common Hookworm (Ankylostoma 1 cm long) is not usually seen in the stools and is diagnosed by finding the eggs using a microscope. If the worms are present in large numbers, they may produce serious effects on the host. They attach themselves to the lining of the small intestine and suck blood, and may cause chronic severe anaemia.

HOOKWORM

Hookworm was recognized in Nyasaland in the early years of this century. In 1909 Livingstonia News reported : "Ankylostoma was more widespread than previously thought." Many people would not have any symptoms but those with heavy infestations were anaemic and had puffy legs.

	Hookworm Surveys	
1913	North Ngara	45% hookworm positive
1930	Nkhota Kota	69% hookworm positive
1930	Zomba	32% hookworm positive

The mode of transmission (as in so many parasites) is bizarre. In 1901, Loess in Cairo accidentally spilled a culture of hookworm larvae on his hands. A dermatitis developed and the hookworm ova were found in his stool. The larvae were able to burrow through the skin (usually of the foot), enter the blood stream and via the heart migrate to the lungs, and then through the throat down to the intestines.

Eucalyptus oil and Beta Naphthol were used as treatment as well as other plant extracts. "Bandawe 1917, the outstanding feature of the medical work this year is the growing popularity of treatment for helminthiasis (worms) for which it has been impossible to keep up an adequate supply of drugs." A more effective drug was found in the 1920s in the U.S.A. Dr.M. Hall observed that patients after chloroform anaesthesia often passed a number of intestinal parasites. Chloroform was too toxic to be used as a worm treatment so other chemicals containing carbon and chlorine were tested. Carbon Tetrachloride $C\ Cl_4$, (chloroform is $CHCl_2$) was found suitable, and if used carefully, relatively safe.

Because of its toxic effect on the liver, patients were told to abstain from alcohol for 3 days before the treatment. Some did not, as Dr.Watson found out at Karonga. A known heavy drinker came for treatment; told the dispenser he had been off beer, and that the Doctor had given permission for him to be treated; all untrue. He was given carbon tetrachloride with the result that he died of acute liver failure. The campaign was stopped and the District Commissioner held a meeting of Chiefs and Councillors. Fortunately for the hookworm campaign, one of the Councillors was able to confirm that the deceased had been drunk in his company the night before he had treatment. Opinion was "the deceased's own foolishness killed him", and they requested the campaign continue.

In the 1930s there were various hookworm campaigns. In the north Dr.Watson treated 4,461 cases. Doses of carbon tetrachloride were given out followed by Epsom salts as a purgative. Between doses, lectures on the various worms and sanitation were given. "The campaign proceeded without a hitch. The people being generally impressed by the quantity of the round worms and tape worms voided after treatment, the hookworms being too small for consideration. Numerous people came from villages further afield asking for treatment and the whole campaign was very popular." Dr.Watson became known as Dr.Chimbudzi (stool)!

In the Lower Shire Dr.Gopsill wrote "the older generation, especially the women, are very conservative and mostly favour native medicine." 150 people were treated and made hookworm free. It was remarkable what a change took place in these infected patients soon after treatment. They noticed increased redness of their mouths, increased appetite, decrease in puffiness of their eyes and feet, and their previous abdominal pains went.

It was inevitable that most of these people would have become reinfected within a short period as few villages had any pit latrines, merely a latrine ground nearby. The idea of "building a little house for my excretions " as one Chief put it, was regarded as laughable, but eventually by persuasion and even by fines for those who did not comply, these "little houses" became common.

In the 1930s, first Blantyre and then Zomba had a daily nightsoil collection, using iron receptacles carried by lorry and the sewerage was emptied into pits. Later, when piped water was installed, a water carriage sewerage system could operate. The construction of the Hynde Dam in Blantyre facilitated a piped water supply in 1930. When this later became inadequate, a scheme to pipe water from the Shire River at Walker Ferry was built in 1963, and has since been enlarged. Lilongwe had piped filtered river water in 1932.

At Fort Manning (Mchinji) in 1932, 11,390 villagers were treated with carbon tetrachloride, 48 pit latrines made and 109 wells cleared. Carbon tetrachloride has long since been superceded by a succession of drugs less toxic and more effective. However in some rural areas only 30% of households have a pit latrine today.

BILHARZIA

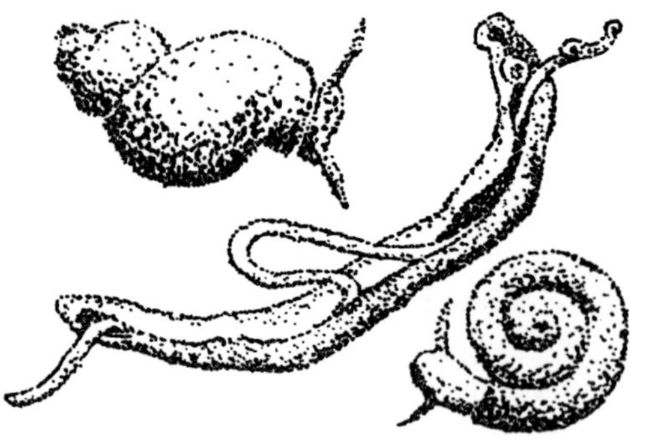

Bilharzia. The fluke is 2cm long. Snails not to scale.

This disease has probably been present for thousands of years in Malaŵi. The Great Lakes are believed to be the cradle of the disease, and bilharzia eggs were found in a 5,000 year old Egyptian mummy. Theodor Bilharz identified the causative worm or fluke in 1852. The life cycle of the fluke through man and snail is very curious but all too common. The adult flukes live in the veins of the abdominal organs of man. They produce eggs which are passed in the urine or stool.

These eggs hatch and the larvae must enter certain varieties of water snail to complete the next stage. Here they multiply and escape from the snail into the water. Anybody in contact with the water may have their skin penetrated by this stage of the larvae, sometimes producing an itchy rash. They enter the blood stream, mature into adults, and continue the cycle.

Livingstone noted blood in the urine in his men from time to time. This is the most common symptom, as the eggs laid by the flukes in the veins of the bladder ulcerate through the lining and are passed in the urine. The severity of the symptoms probably depends on the load of flukes that the patient carries. The liver and kidney are also affected. There are two types of the disease in Malaŵi, Schistosoma haematobium which affects mainly the bladder, which is ten times more prevalent than Schistosoma mansoni, which affects the bowel. Schistosoma, meaning split body (the female encloses the male), is the name of the fluke.

Thousands of people live with these parasites (as with hookworm and malaria) all their lives, developing a sort of immunity, and coping with the loss of blood and other minor complications. No doubt it contributes to ill health, even if they do not develop major complications of kidney or liver damage, or bladder carcinoma. The high incidence of bladder cancer in the country is related to this disease.

Dr.Howard estimated in the early 1900s that 50% of the Lakeshore population was affected with the majority in good health. In 1929, Dr.Gopsill in the Lower Shire Valley found 70% of 100 apparently fit men had S.haematobium infection, by finding the typical eggs in their urine. Antimony tartrate was being given intravenously as a treatment in 1918, and by 1923 the UMCA reports queues of patients waiting for treatment.

In 1940 41% of soldiers in the King's African Rifles were found to be infected. At this time Dr.Ransford found that 51% of children were infected in Nkhota Kota, but interestingly that the incidence in adults was less, indicating that a degree of immunity developed, or the severely affected children had died.

New treatments were developed; Nilodin, then Ambilhar, although all with some side effects. Reinfection was almost certain in every case unless strict and often impractical hygienic measures were taken.

In 1949, 10,000 cases were recorded as being treated, probably a pale reflection of the total number of cases. Ten years later in the Lower Shire 15,445 cases were reported,"although this in no way represents the true incidence; chronic complications of the disease are widespread; cancer of the bladder, chronic

> *Sir,*
>
> *This is at midnight of the dated. I have woke up because I cannot sleep. Life looses its meaning with a lot of S. haematobium larvae and eggs in my blood vessels. Why keep on living? or am I to survive and live on taking some kinds of pills every fortnight when I feel the disease is tough on me? My hopes are failing in vain. Shall I ever get married, sure not in my present condition? These are some of the questions I can't answer when the haematobium is tough on me.*
>
> *The abdomen bubbling, like little african women are doing their pounding business there. The pain extended through the belly muscles reaching somewhere to the area of the heart is like a needle fixed in there to patrol this specified field. The metrifonate was defeated may be the very day I took it! But now what is remaining? Am I waiting to meet my doom where I should retire and join those who are spending their days below the surface of the earth where there is no sunbathing in a morning of a cold winter.*
>
> A moving extract from a letter to a Blantyre Doctor 1984

pyelonephritis with hydronephrosis is a frequent finding. It is the most incapacitating disease in the Lower Shire Valley." In 1961, 24,825 cases were treated.

As is found elsewhere in the world where irrigation schemes are set up, the snails followed the canals and the disease incidence increased. This was so in the Lower Shire and at Dwangwa on the Lakeshore where there are sugar plantations. At Dwangwa, 40% of those surveyed were infected. In 1980 it was estimated there were 2 million cases in the country (200 million worldwide), ranging from 50% to 15% of the population depending on the area.

There have been improvements in treatment over the past ten years, drugs involving fewer side effects and greater efficacy have been developed. Praziquantel is now the (expensive) drug of choice. Efforts at controlling snail populations have only met with partial success. Reinfection remains almost certain for most of the affected populations. The tourist beaches around the Lake which are free of reeds are reasonably safe from the risk of the disease.

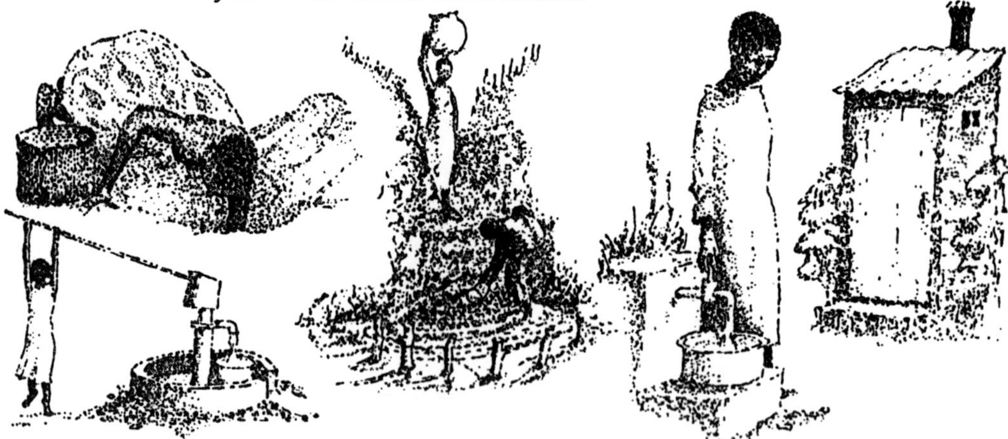

Water and Sanitation, more important than medicines. Digging in a dry steam bed; bore hole pump; stake protection against crocodiles, Shire River; protected spring; improved latrine.

In June 1891, Dr.Sorabji Boyce from Bombay was appointed as the first Government doctor. Within six months he was killed at Kisungulu by Chief Makanjila's men. He had courageously gone ashore from the British gunboat *Domira* to retrieve the body of Captain Maguire, when he accompanied the military expedition against the slave traders on the east shore of Lake Nyasa.

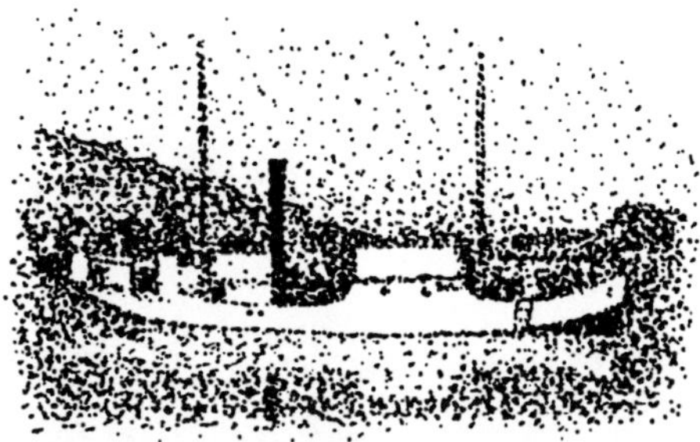

Domira

By the end of the century, the Government was employing a few physicians in addition to the naval doctors on the British anti -slavery gunboats which patrolled the Lake. Government medical services were centred at Zomba, with outstations at Nkhota Kota, Karonga, and Chiromo. In 1896 the first proper government hospital in Nyasaland was built at Zomba. For many years though, most areas had no hospitals.

The "Outfit of Medical Officers proceeding to British Central Africa" in 1898 envisaged a doctor on 'ulendo', touring the country with porters carrying his equipment, and sleeping in a tent at night. He was advised to bring a tent, bed, mosquito net, and cooking utensils; a hypodermic syringe, set of dental instruments, pocket surgical instrument set with forceps, scalpels, sutures, needles, silk, catheters, amputating case, and ophthalmic case. Also he had to bring a supply of drugs, including arsenic, quinine, and morphia.

One such doctor commented "I visited every corner of Nyasaland: there were no roads, only hoed native paths, and no transport. It was a wonderful country." One advantage of these bush doctors was that they could observe the entire disease environment, and make scientific observations of the factors involved. At the turn of the century, measures to control and prevent disease became possible.These are described in other chapters and include these following projects:

In 1898 the British Government with the Royal Society sent a research commission on malaria and blackwater fever to Nyasaland, to study the distribution of the anopheles mosquito.

In 1904 a systematic vaccination campaign of the general population was begun, with local vaccinators and lymph paid for by the Government. This abated subsequent smallpox epidemics.

ZOMBA. OCTOBER 15, 1896.

I. LAMAGNA & CO.

Drugs, Medicines and Toilet Requisites Department.

Customers and the public in general are hereby informed that this

DEPARTMENT

is now well assorted. Orders will be thankfully received, and promptly and carefully executed.

OINTMENTS:—Carbolic, Holloway's, Eczema Cream.

TONICS:—Iron and Quinine, Clark's Blood Mixture and Liver Tonic, Sarsaparilla, Cod Liver Oil, Beef and Malt Wine.

QUININE:—5 gr. and 2 gr. tabloids; powder, ½oz. bottle.

PILLS:—Carter's Little Liver Pills, Livingstone Rousers, Bronchial Troches, Pine-tar Lozenges, Geraudel's Pastilles, Iodine.

Essence of Rennet; Pure Glycerine in bottles.
People's Embrocation; Ellimam's Embrocation; Homocea.
Camphor Tablets. Trusses.
Thermometers—Clinical Thermometers.

TOILET REQUISITES:—Tooth Brushes, Carbolic Tooth Pastes, Eucalyptus, Cherry, Areca Nut Tooth Pastes.

Pommades, Cosmetiques, assorted.

Brushes:—Tooth, Hair, Shaving and Nail Brushes.
Razors, Razor Strops, Oil Stones.

Bay Rum, Triple Orange Flower Water; Elder Flower Water; Eau de Cologne, Alcohol de Menthe.

SPONGE BAGS, TOOTH BRUSH BAGS.

Pears' Unscented Soaps, Pears' Transparent Glycerine Soap, Pears' Transparent Soap Balls, Pears' Shaving Sticks.

FILTERS:—Silicated Carbon Filters, Maignen's Filters. Gazogenes

Dr.Eldred surveyed hookworm in Karonga, Fort Johnston, and Zomba, in 1912 finding that about 30% of people were then infested. The need for pit latrines was emphasized.

The sleeping sickness epidemic led to drastic measures to control tsetse flies in 1912.

Dr.G.M.Sanderson surveyed filariasis along the banks of the Ruo River in 1912, finding 27% of persons infected, and the control of mosquitoes was needed.

Dr.Hugh Stannus(1905-14), worked at Zomba: "We took our own microscopes, and everything cried out to be observed, collected, and noted." Enthusiastically he did a helminthic survey, made a collection of parasitic worms from man, reptiles, and mammals, and did hundreds of collections of human blood parasites. He diagnosed the first indigenous case of sleeping sickness in Nyasaland at Nkhota Kota. He identified East Coast fever in cattle here.

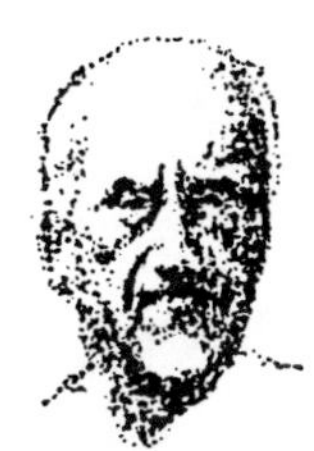

Dr.Stannus

In 1910 -11, Dr.Stannus observed "a number of cases of skin eruptions among the inmates of Zomba Central Prison", which, after further careful study, enabled him to make a diagnosis of pellagra (vitamin B deficiency). With the exception of Robben Island, this was the first time this disease had been observed in Africa. Stannus noted that the rash occurred on parts of the body exposed to the sun, especially the lips. He was able to establish that this pellagra was due to deficient diet at the prison (1½ lbs.of rice per day). He also found pellagra patients in local villages. By 1915, the Government noted "the marked decline in pellagra since the introduction of an improved diet in Zomba Prison is noteworthy". Dr.Stannus' scientific work led to improvements far beyond the prison. He built the first pathology laboratory in the country, he started the first medical library, and he published papers on pellagra, sleeping sickness, piroplasmosis in dogs, helminths, albinism, congenital deformities, tropical diseases, and blackwater fever. He departed in 1914, when he enlisted in the King's African Rifles to go to Tanganyika.

Dr.J.B.Davey, medical officer at Dedza in 1912, set out to examine all 5,815 people living in villages between the Lake and Dedza Hills. He was looking for sleeping sickness, but in his report he noted many other conditions: 93% of the people bore marks of smallpox, goitre caused by iodine deficiency was common, yaws was endemic and very serious, old fractures and injuries were very evident, several cases of leprosy were diagnosed, syphilis was a problem, there was no tuberculosis, and elephantiasis which was common at Karonga, did not occur on this southern lakeshore.

In 1914, Government hospital facilities in Nyasaland were still minimal.

Hospital Beds 1914	
Port Herald	4
Blantyre	12
Zomba	46
Fort Johnston	6
Karonga	2

The 1914-18 War put more strains on the medical services, money from Europe was limited for a decade afterwards. Seven of the twelve doctors employed by Government were called up into the army, to go to Tanganyika. 169,000 carriers were employed in the First World War. Seven major carrier hospitals, each in charge of a doctor, were set up; (see Sr.Jacques in the Catholic chapter). With depleted resources, Services were continued.

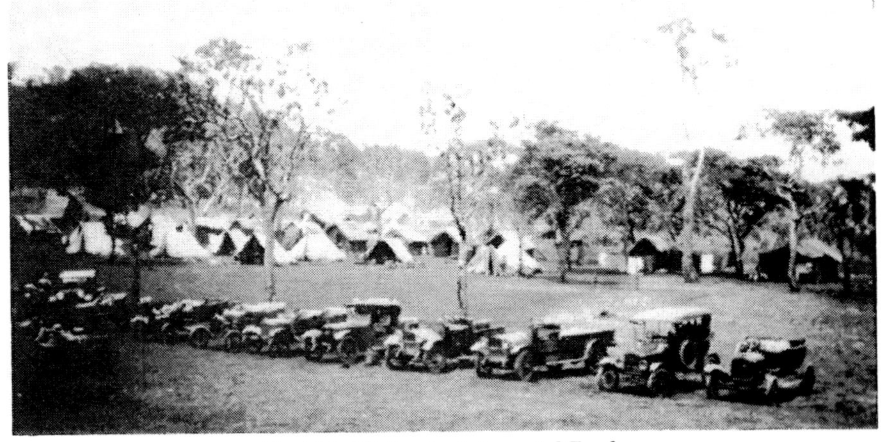

First World War; tented hospital, Zomba.

At the end of 1918 the global pandemic of influenza reached the country. Special hospitals were set up. More than 60 Europeans (including 2 military doctors), and an unknown number of Africans died (the recorded figure was 1,683). A severe smallpox epidemic was contained in 1915, continual vigilance over sleeping sickness was maintained, and big anti-rat measures prevented the spread of bubonic plague in 1917. A bad drought caused famine in Nyasaland in 1922. The first Lilongwe hospital was built then on the site of the Golf Club; it was later described: "the native hospital at Lilongwe is built of temporary materials and is beyond repair."

In these difficult conditions, 135 Medical Dressers trained to perform some routine proceedures, were very successful in attracting more village people to seek medical care, instead of going to the witch doctor. Government Reports for 1925 stated "the increase in the number of outpatients is chiefly due to the increasing work of the 78 rural dispensaries. These dispensaries are built of sundried mud bricks with thatched roofs." These Medical Dressers demonstrated the need for African trained medical staff to challenge ignorance, poverty, and disease.

Difficult conditions prevailed in many hospitals. Dr.Watson described Karonga in 1926: "Patients arrived at the hospital by canoe across the Lake, which was more comfortable than being carried in a jolting machila(hammock on a pole). Hospital buildings were very primitive. If a doctor was willing to turn builder, it was amazing what could be achieved with a small grant of funds. I built an operating room with a sterilizing room, and ward of four beds attached. Karonga hospital consisted of a two room brick dispensary, a brick thatched building of four small wards, and another building for 10 leprosy patients. The beds were made locally with stretched ox hides as mattresses. I went to the bush to select trees to be felled to make furniture for the rural dispensaries."

Outpatients (new patients)			
1922	1923	1924	1926
39,313	96,088	114,043	116,140

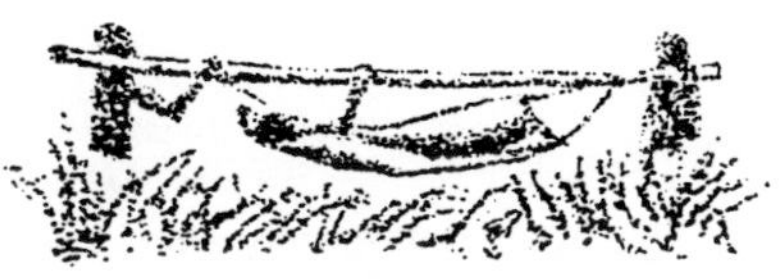

Machila

By 1929 a poor picture of Government hospitals was given: "Fort Manning (Mchinji): the hospital is built of temporary materials, and is now in a dilapidated state beyond repair." At Chikwawa "the hospital consists of wattle and daub huts except for a very small dispensary made of bricks and iron, 55 patients were admitted during the year. There are 4 rural dispensaries, 3 built of wattle and one of bricks with a thatched roof. Between them they attended 3,710 patients. An Indian sub-assistant surgeon is in charge."

In 1930, following the Shircore Report, (Dr.Owen Shircore had worked in Nyasaland previously), £78,284 was provided from the Colonial Development Fund in Britain to build new hospitals.

These new hospitals were all completed by 1934			
Hospital beds			
Zomba	100	Nkhota Kota	50
Mulanje	50	Mzimba	30
Thyolo	50	Karonga	50
Chikwawa	30	Mchinji	30
Chiradzulu	30		
Lilongwe	30		
Dowa	30		
Kasungu	30		

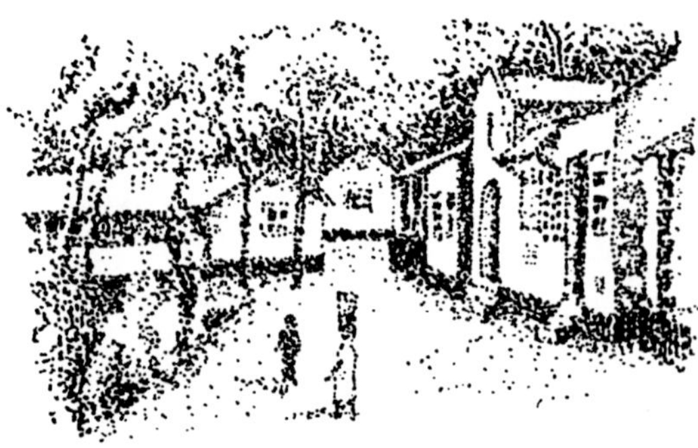

Old or Bottom Hospital, Lilongwe today.

Extra wards were built at Fort Johnston, Port Herald, and Dedza. The number of hospital beds was increased from 170 to 634. This was one bed per 2,500 persons (the League of Nations ideal was one bed per 1,000 persons).

Then other problems arose: "It is unfortunate that most of the hospitals remain half empty". However, a good surgical and medical service soon attracted patients, and these hospitals were later crowded. By the mid 1930s, there was a doctor or sub-assistant surgeon in charge of 15 of the 20 district headquarters.

At the outbreak of World War II, 10 out of 18 Government doctors joined the army, 24 medical dressers were seconded to the military. African Hospital Assistants now successfully took charge of 8 hospitals. The first Specialist Surgeon, Mr. M.A.W. Roberts F.R.C.S. came to Nyasaland in 1942, and new operating theatres with electric sterilizers were opened at Zomba.

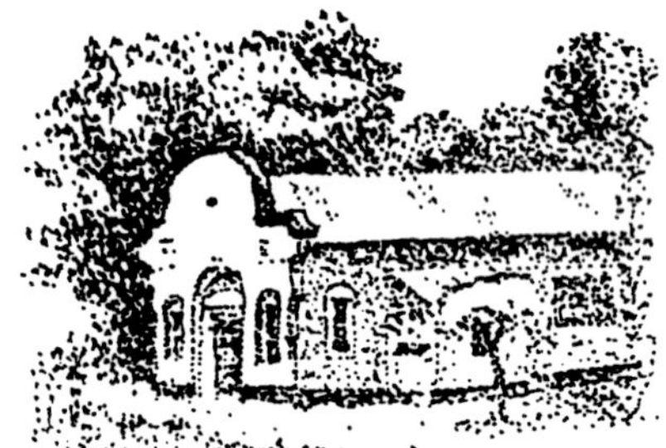

Part of Zomba Hospital.

The post-war years were ones of severe financial limitations. The rural dispensaries were dilapidated, drugs were in short supply, there was just enough sulphone for the leprosaria, and streptomycin for the TB patients was a priority, but there was not enough penicillin to treat sexually transmitted diseases and arsenicals were still used in 1951.

In difficult conditions, local medical staff were trained and two Specialist Surgeons and a Physician appointed. Specialist services quickly caused an increase in the demand for hospital care. By 1950 "In the Government African Hospitals there are 1,115 beds...daily average inpatient state was 1,157, and despite an increased turnover of patients, it is now essential to provide more accommodation in African Hospitals." The population of Nyasaland was 2·5 million in 1950, and programmes to treat and control leprosy, malaria, filariasis, yaws, and smallpox, had begun.

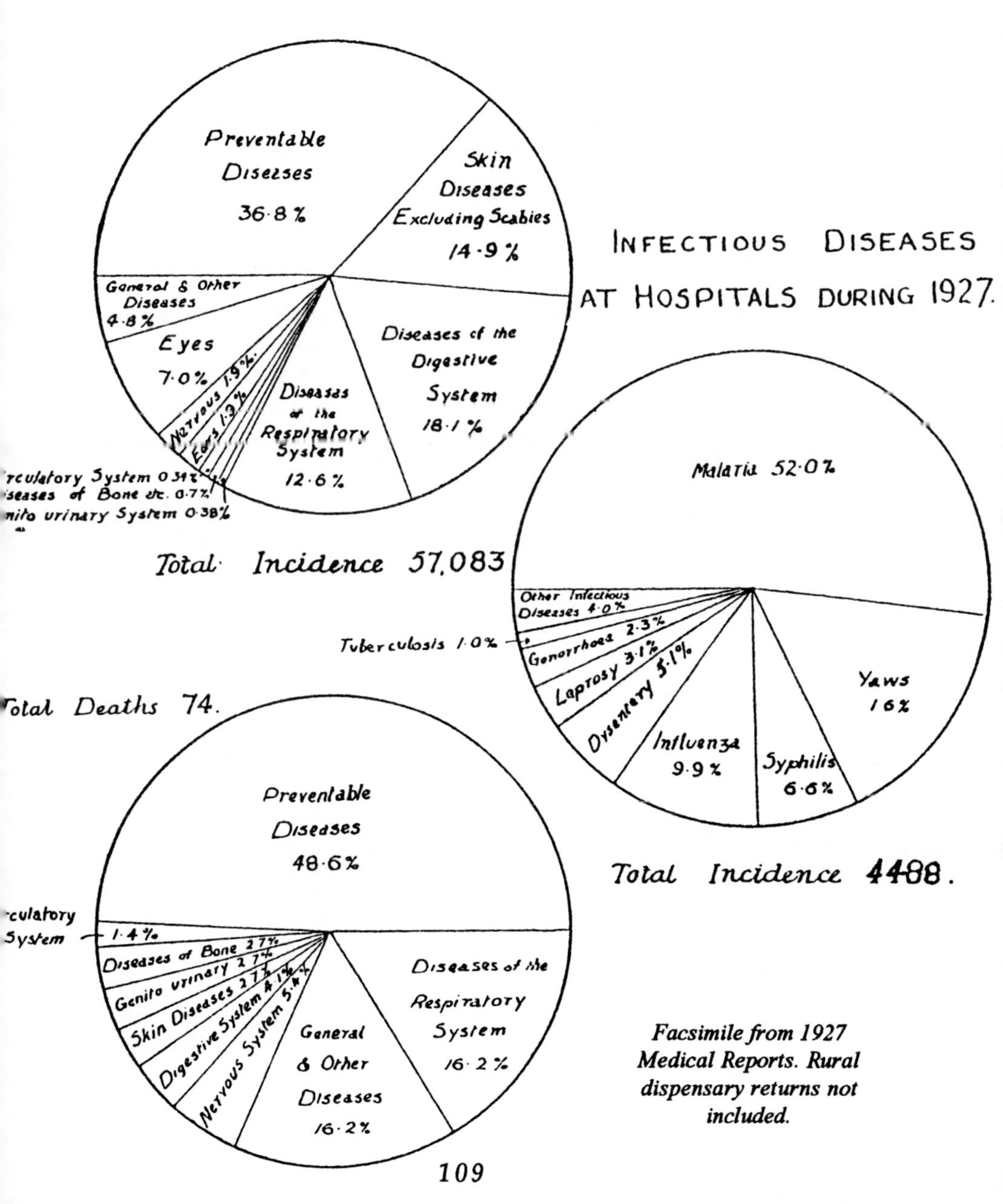

The Proportion of Preventable, Systemic and other Diseases shown as Percentages of Total Cases treated at Hospitals during 1927.
Preventable Diseases 36.8 %
Skin Diseases Excluding Scabies 14.9 %
General & Other Diseases 4.8 %
Eyes 7.0 %
Nervous 1.9 %
Ears 1.3 %
Diseases of the Respiratory System 12.6 %
Diseases of the Digestive System 18.1 %
Circulatory System 0.34 %
Diseases of Bone etc. 0.7 %
Genito urinary System 0.38 %
Total Incidence 57,083
INFECTIOUS DISEASES AT HOSPITALS DURING 1927.
Malaria 52.0 %
Other Infectious Diseases 4.0 %
Tuberculosis 1.0 %
Gonorrhoea 2.3 %
Leprosy 3.1 %
Dysentery 3.1 %
Influenza 9.9 %
Syphilis 6.6 %
Yaws 16 %
Total Incidence 4488.
Total Deaths 74.
Preventable Diseases 48.6 %
Circulatory System 1.4 %
Diseases of Bone 2.7 %
Genito urinary 2.7 %
Skin Diseases 2.7 %
Digestive System 4.1 %
Nervous System 5.4 %
General & Other Diseases 16.2 %
Diseases of the Respiratory System 16.2 %
Facsimile from 1927 Medical Reports. Rural dispensary returns not included.

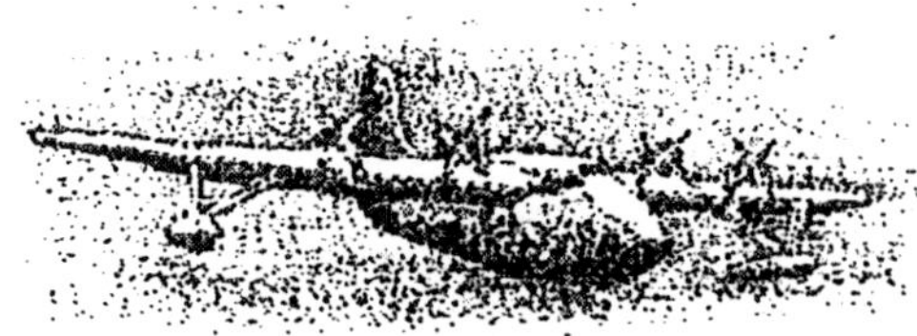

Short Solent Flying Boat. Cape Maclear 1950

During the Colonial era, a pioneering first aid service, was slowly developed to become a comprehensive modern medical service, offering specialist facilities in central hospitals, medical care in all district hospitals, and health care in rural clinics. During this period psychiatric services were developed by government at Zomba. Without the economic problems created by two World Wars, progress might have been more rapid. The medical service established by 1952 was the foundation of the service today.

ZOMBA MENTAL HOSPITAL

The most important mental illnesses seen are acute disturbances due to physical illness (organic psychoses due to meningitis or typhoid), or alchohol, or chamba (marihuana); schizophrenia (dissociation from reality), and manic depressive psychoses (abnormal swings of mood). Today there are effective drugs but it was not always so. When proper records were started in 1919 in Zomba, most of the patients were classified as Criminal Lunatics and the Asylum was run on penal lines. There were 30 patients and some had been there for 10 years. The medical officer from the prison half a mile away would visit occasionally.

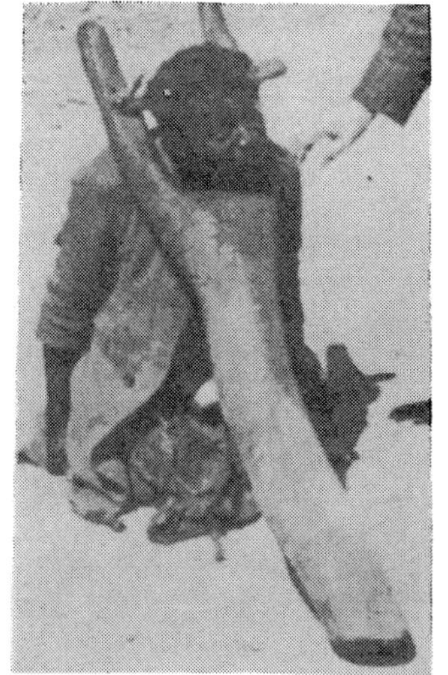

Village restraint on a mentally disturbed man. Dedza area, 1950's.

In the 1930s improvements were made but inmates were confined to cells and often manacled. In 1950 the Governor ordered new pavilion type wards to be built, and a Medical Officer and Hospital Assistant were appointed. There were 150 patients, 16 female. Most were schizophrenic. It was felt that there were fewer manic depressive patients than in a comparable European institution. The controlled use of sedatives (phenobarbitone and paraldehyde) produced a great improvement in the previously noisy and disturbed atmosphere. Patients' nutrition improved and they were allowed to do some casual work. Electro-convulsive therapy was started with beneficial results.

Later in the 1950s powerful drugs were developed that could control the patient's moods. Some had a calming action, Largactil being the best known, and some were anti-depressant or allayed anxiety.

In the late 1960s, nurses were sent to Britain for psychiatric training, and they have since formed the basis of mental care in Malaŵi. There has only occasionally been a Specialist Psychiatrist in the country. In 1982, Enrolled Psychiatric Nurses were trained locally. Recently they have been posted to District hospitals. Patients now have the opportunity of treatment in their home areas, and the previously overcrowded Mental Hospital now has a more manageable 250 patients; there is a new children's ward.

Mental illness is usually seen as the sphere of the Traditional Healer, but the public are gradually becoming aware that Western Medicine has much to offer, and that disturbed patients can be restored to society.

FOOD

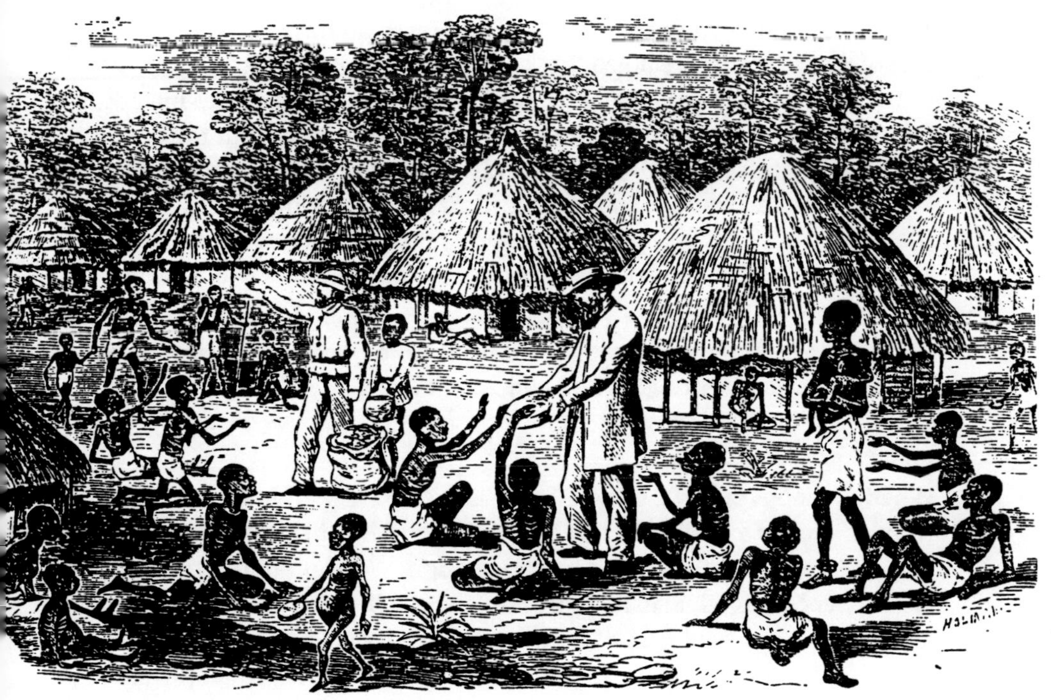

The Famine. "Disease accompanies this insufficient supply of food and a stomach illness which Rowley could not arrest, carried off a considerable number of our children." (Christmas Day, Magomero 1861)

In the late 1930s here were several nutritional surveys including the detailed Platt Report.Some of the findings are valid today, and it is interesting to make some comparisons with the present situation.

The pre-war surveys found relatively few dietary taboos, and in the days before the population increase, most smallholder farmers had enough land to grow food to last the whole year. Today many plots have been so sub-divided that a member of the extended family has to seek employment to buy maize meal. The harvest will depend on fertilizer in the depleted soil and not all can afford this. In the early hungry months of the year, before the crop is ready, when the 'nkhokwe' stores are almost empty, luckily the mangoes are in season. This delicious fruit, introduced from Asia, is eaten in large quantities, often more than 10 a day. Many people's palms of the hands and soles of the feet turn yellow, a harmless side effect.

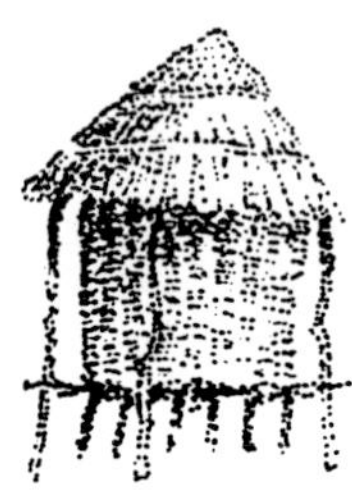

Nkhokwe

Maize is prepared as porridge, nsima, in different ways. The coarsely ground 'ngaiwa' contains more bran, protein, and fat, than the more refined 'ufa'. One of the early surveys noted that prisoners in Zomba fed on ngaiwa, often put on weight in spite of hard labour. An attempt was made to introduce this more nutritious, but less liked nsima into the hospital, but the patients were greatly upset and ufa was quickly re-introduced. The local maize is white and when some donated yellow maize was brought in at a time of shortage, it was not acceptable. Throughout the world, dietary habits are learnt early and changed only with difficulty. Maize eaters will be reluctant to take Cassava nsima.

Cassava, is an important crop, introduced from South America 300 years ago. It is resistant to drought, and will grow in inferior soil. Since 1970 mealy bug infestation has reduced yields and local research is currently being undertaken to combat this.

Whether maize, cassava, or rice, is the staple food, depending on the region, wood is needed to cook it. This is becoming very short in many areas, women having to walk long distances to find enough. Wood planting schemes are actively encouraged, usually with Blue Gums. The old hardwood trees are fast disappearing having been used for furniture or charcoal making.

Whatever the staple diet, a relish, 'ndiwo', is needed.This may be meat or fish, but for many these are occasional luxuries. Beans, fungi, groundnuts, rodents, flying termites, are more often used to provide additional protein and added flavour. Also important is salt; either bought, leached from the soil, or water made salty by filtering through ash from various plants, often banana stems, papyrus, or other grasses. One 1930s survey pointed out that the local beer made from millet, sorghum, or maize, contains a lot of solids and can be considered a nutritious food, in moderation!

Vetinary efforts in the 1930s improved the quality and supply of meat; this included dipping to combat tick borne East Coast Fever, and castration of scrub bulls. In 1936, 1,200 cattle were exported from the North to the goldfields at Lupa in Tanganyika.

Then, as now, there were considerable losses, due to flies, of dried and smoked fish. Research is proceeding on ways of preventing this. It is estimated that up to one third of foodstuffs is spoiled in storage. The use of modern insecticides, when affordable, has improved yields and decreased these losses.

As in much of the rest of Africa, the food production per capita is decreasing, and not keeping pace with the population growth. Malnourished people are more likely to fall ill and die than those with an adequate diet.

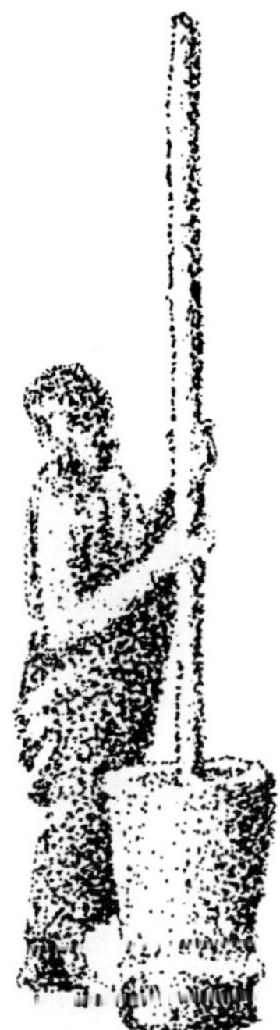

Pounding Maize.

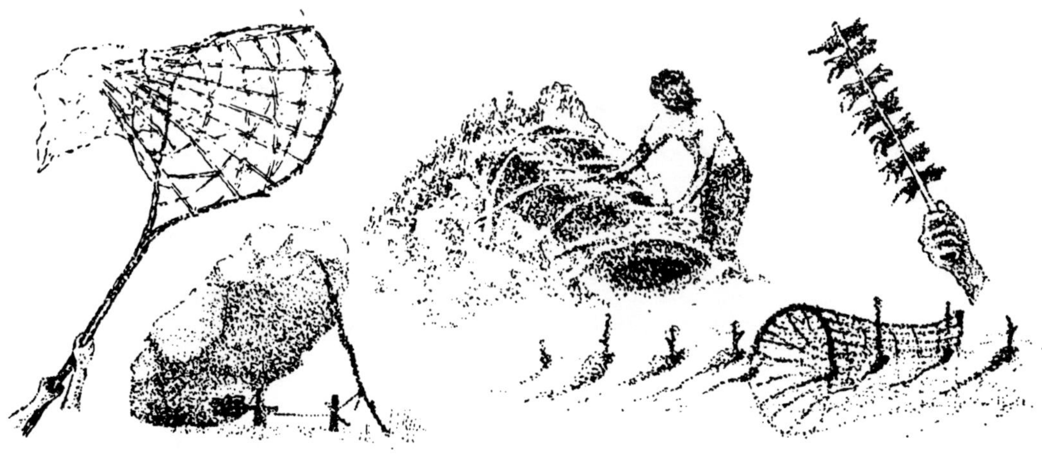

Extra protein for some. Net for bats; small rodent trap; flying termites trap, a basin of water is put at the bottom; fish trap in a weir made from branches; mice for sale.

17   SLEEPING SICKNESS

In the 16th century from the New World came reports of a mysterious lethargy that fell on slaves from certain parts of Africa. Slaves would fall sick in the West Indies, this was attributed to home sickness, but may have been Sleeping Sickness. In the early 1900s, the number of cases of Sleeping Sickness in the Congo and Uganda started to increase. Within a few years the population around Lake Victoria was reduced by a third. A commission from Britain went to investigate in 1902. One of the members, Castellani, found a single celled organism, a trypanosome, in the cerebro-spinal fluid of patients. It was not immediately realized that these were the cause of this disease, until Sir David Bruce defined the situation. He had previously worked on 'Nagana', a trypanosome disease of cattle in South Africa.

The Nyasaland Government was worried that this disease might spread south to them in miners returning from Katanga. Commissions including entomologists were set up, and increased funds were made available. The river tsetse, Glossina Palpalis, was known to transmit the trypanosome from buck to man, but this fly was not found in the country. The bush tsetse, Glossina Morsitans was however found, and it was possible it could spread the disease. Tsetse flies have their mouth parts permanently pointing forward from the head, and at rest their wings overlap.

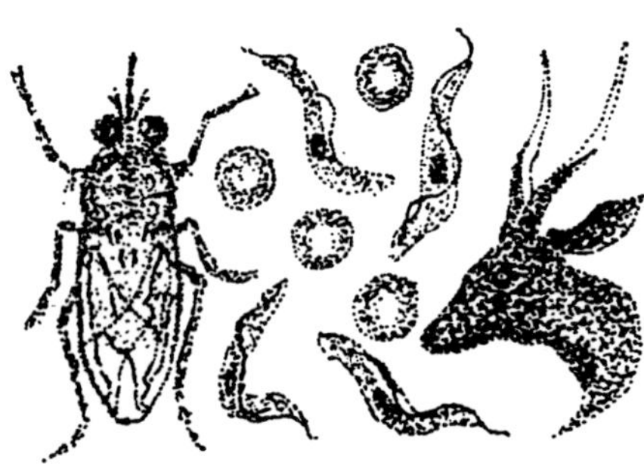

Buck, tsetse fly and magnified trypanasomes among red blood cells.

In 1907 a special post was set up at Karonga to screen travellers entering the country. The next year Dr.Davey confirmed Sleeping Sickness by finding the trypanosomes in the fluid from enlarged neck glands in a patient. The victim had however been to Tanganyika so he may have acquired the disease there. He was segregated in a special camp at Ngani Hill in Dowa district. One year later Dr.Stannus confirmed this disease in Nkhota Kota in a patient who had never left the country.

Captain Dr.Hardy, in charge of West Nyasa district, succumbed to Sleeping Sickness. He was treated with Atoxyl injections, a toxic arsenical drug which produced blindness and did not improve his condition. He was invalided out but died in Aden in 1909 on his way home. In 1910, Dr.W.A.Murray at

Mvera also confirmed a case in an African who had never left the country. He found trypanosomes in the blood of members of a South African hunting party touring Mvera area, as well. It was becoming clear that G.Morsitans might be the vector. This was confirmed in 1912 by Kinghorn and York* in Luangwa, and confirmed by Bruce working with his cages of monkeys at Kasu, near Mvera.

Between 1909 and 1911, there were 42 new cases. Active measures were taken. Special locally trained Reporters of Sickness carried out surveys and took blood smears. Sleeping Sickness Police ensured the clearance of bushes around villages and along main roads where tsetse flies would settle. Latrines were built in clearings to prevent the bush being used for this purpose. Game was destroyed, "clear out the game and you clear out the tsetse" (Dr.Prentice).

Dr.Davey reported an unusual attempt to control this fly. Koch, of tuberculosis fame, had a theory that tsetse flies feed on crocodile blood (not true). "The authorities offered 3d for a crocodile egg. A headman of North Nyasa district asked for a weekend off and returned on the

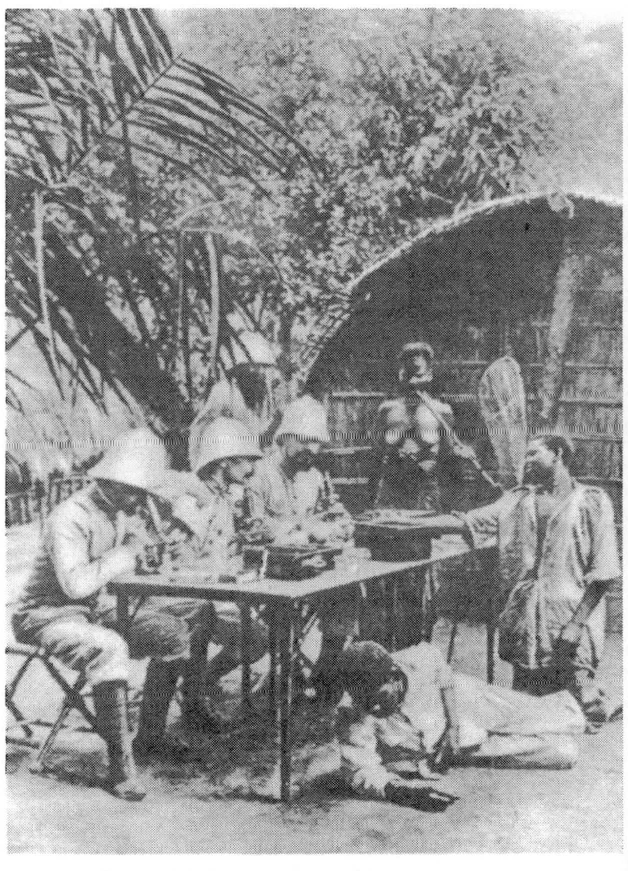

1906 Sleeping Sickness Survey. Koch facing camera

Monday morning, followed by a string of women with baskets on their heads. They contained 8,000 eggs. The price of crocodile eggs was promptly reduced".

For a while the Livingstonia Mission post on the Fort Jameson -Serenje road (N.Rhodesia) had a steady income examining several hundreds of travellers into the country at 2/6 a time. The road was later closed. By 1913 there had been 163 confirmed cases of Sleeping Sickness, but it was also becoming

* *Illus. inside front cover*

clear that they were different from the Ugandan and West African ones. The disease was a smouldering type with a small steady death rate, instead of the devastating epidemic type seen there. The trypanosomes looked a little different and were labelled T.Rhodesiense as opposed to T. Gambiense.

Dr.Wigan, Nkhota Kota, 1913: "A monitor in one of our schools was sent for dressings for a swelling at the back of his neck, a sign of trypanosomiasis. I found he had microbes for Sleeping Sickness in his blood. He lived until nearly the end of the year." After the end of World War I, the entomologist Lamborn continued investigations including attempts to breed parasites in a colony of blowflies that could be used to control tsetse.

Sporadic cases continued to be reported. In 1931 there were 10 patients in Nkhota Kota. In 1940 there were 7 cases, from Mzimba, Nkhota Kota, and Fort Johnston. By the end of the Second World War the development of residual insecticides, DDT, Gammexane, gave new hope of destroying the tsetse fly. The main fly belt was Dowa, Dedza, Mangochi, Liwonde. Vehicles going through the fly belts had to enter a barn and be sprayed, or workers with nets would inspect and catch flies in cars.

It was expensive and not simple, and today the use of insecticides is concentrated on either spraying in very carefully controlled doses and droplet size from aircraft; or in the use of traps, usually large sheets of dark material impregnated with insecticide and baited with chemicals, mimicking the odour of cattle.

Cases continue to be reported. In 1953, after some years absence, Sleeping Sickness reappeared in Chikwawa. In 1984, 21 patients were admitted to Rumphi hospital. A survey of villages in the Vwaza Marsh area showed a 4·2% trypanosome positive smear. Other cases have been reported recently from Mangochi and Nkhota Kota, related to game parks.

There are more effective, although still toxic, treatments for the disease today, and it is unlikely that Malaŵi will experience the devastating epidemics that occurred in Zaire in 1960 or Uganda in 1980.

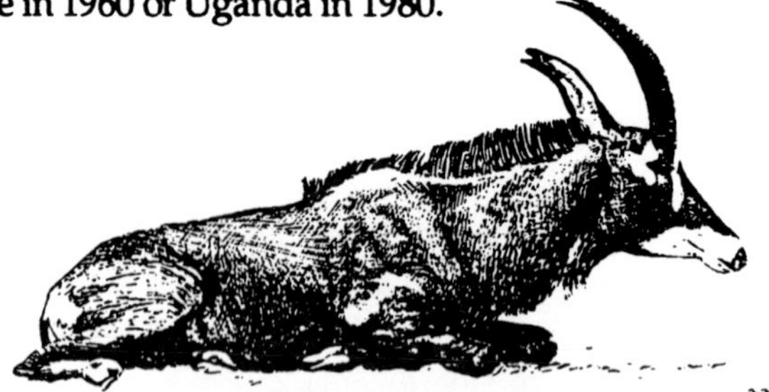

Roan Antelope. Drawn by Sir H.Johnston

18   DR. and MRS. GEORGE PRENTICE
(served 1894-1924)

The Church of Scotland sent George Prentice L.R.C.P.and M.R.C.S. (Edin) to take charge of Bandawe Mission upon the departure of Dr.Laws to Kondowe in 1894. He wrote "speak of a hospital and you were told no African would sleep in a room in which another had died. The first death in a hospital would close its doors." His keen interest in medicine soon made him busy in the Bandawe dispensary: "it is the oldest building still standing, it still serves its purpose, though erected in 1880 of wattle and daub." In these conditions he did some remarkable work.

Bandawe 1897 "On December 16th some men arrived, carrying a boy whose right arm had been so badly crushed by a crocodile that gangrene had set in.. we amputated it...he is now getting along nicely." In 1898 he reported "the building is entirely adequate for the needs of medical and surgical work: 16 chloroform cases; two fatty tumours, operated twice for liver abscess, removed tumour weighing 4.75 ounces from the upper eyelid of a woman." He was modest: "two cases puzzled me and made me wish I had spent more time in hospital when at home. I have refused two big operations I was asked to undertake, because I feel unfit to tackle one, and fear the other would not yield the desired result."

By 1900 "the medical work under Dr.Prentice has been fruitful. Some 12,000 cases have been treated this year. Increasing need is felt for proper hospital accommodation." His gynaecological work was noteworthy. Half a century before African women were willing to seek either maternity or gynaecological care (not even from female staff), George Prentice had a thriving practice at Bandawe. In 1897 he performed "a major gynaecological operation, and several minor ones. There is a pretty good field for gynaecology and Tuesday has now been set apart for diseases of women." He actually built the first maternity ward in Nyasaland, which remained empty after he left Bandawe.

The Chewa people at Kasungu had asked for Scottish missionaries to be sent to them, and a local mission station was opened there in 1894. Then, in 1900 George Prentice moved from Bandawe: "we had to spend 10 days getting his belongings packed and away to his new station at Kasungu." He bought a Chewa hut at Chilanga for 3 shillings as his first home: "during the year I have travelled about a good deal in search of timber for use in the permanent buildings, and also to choose centres for outstations...our dwelling house was first put up, the mud walls of wattle and daub were dry enough to allow the house being occupied."

He married in June 1901, and a daughter was born to them at Kasungu in December 1902. "A singing class, conducted by Mrs.Prentice has been of great interest to our more advanced pupils, and choir membership has grown to 50. Mrs.Prentice has also been training the girls in homecraft." She is described as a busy mother and teacher. "She cared for the Station school, and for the large staff of African teachers, helping them greatly when they came for their annual periods of instruction at the central station."

Dr.Prentice pioneered medical work at Kasungu. He wrote in 1902: "Medical work has not been pushed owing to lack of medicines and accommodation, however no needy case has been turned away. One worst case: a lion bit a man who was in a party driving it away from a cow, and he sustained compound fractures in the arm in two places....when he was brought into the Station, we took great pains to have him properly attended to. Next day, to my great disgust, I found the sling in which his arm had been put converted into a loin cloth, while an officious relative endeavoured to hold the broken limb in position now the sling was removed."

By 1903 he had established 6 dispensaries with 2,668 patients in the year in Kasungu district. "I have not as yet commenced charging Africans for medical attention, although I sometimes get small presents." "During a tour through some villages, I saw quite a number of cases suitable for hospital treatment, but we have no inpatient accommodation...my own inclination is to develop this department." In 1906 the mission council passed a resolution to build the hospital as a self help project in Kasungu. Within three years, 200,000 bricks were made and a hospital of two blocks each 76 by 17 feet, was built and roofed.

However Dr.Prentice still continued his district visits and commented on ulendo, "it is wiser to leave the outlying villages until the dry season, then one can feed one's caravan mainly by means of one's rifle, not so in the wet season." In 1910 he diagnosed the first case of Sleeping Sickness at Kasungu, and he wrote tersely about the preservation of wildlife:" One might say that a huge culture medium is being prepared under the protection of European powers or European Sportsmen for the spread of trypanosomiasis ...the protection of game, and the consequent spreading of tsetse with Sleeping Sickness threatening this country, is about as sane a policy as the protection of rats when bubonic plague is threatening a home community."

Within five years the epidemic spread, and the road to Tamanda was impassable with tsetse flies: "if Sleeping Sickness attacks other stations equally virulently, either the whole population will have to be moved, or we will move it on the spot...I was told of a 20% incidence in one district. One of our certificated teachers fell victim." He regarded this man, Noa, as a martyr to the government policy of game protection.

However the Prentices did not retreat. The mission reported in 1914: "the arrival back of Dr.and Mrs.Prentice with their two children was a happy event." A visitor described the Prentice home in 1915: "The house is set on a rise: at Kasungu House you sit on a verandah like the deck of a liner. You look across miles and miles of plain with hills dotted here and there. It is a land flowing with milk and marmalade. This

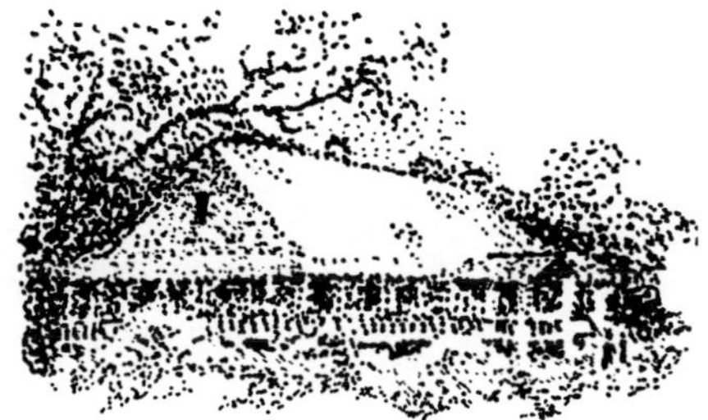

The Prentice's House.

Ngara district is a good centre for hunting, and it has recently been opened to free shooting as a tsetse fly experiment. If you elect to spend your holiday hunting, everything is before you, from the lordly elephant to the wild dog; every kind of antelope, from the Eland to the Pookoo. This Free Shooting concession is largely due to agitation by Dr.Prentice against tsetse flies...the fame of Sing'anga Prentice has spread far. An African from Rhodesia came for help for his fast failing sight, and recently a donkey's blood was tested for trypanosomes, with a positive result."

George Prentice was a keen pathologist. After his first microscope arrived in 1912, he wrote "operative work is perhaps the most gratifying in which the medical missionary can engage; but the laboratory, where he can make messes with Methylene Blue, and, in the region of infinitesimals, with the zest of a schoolboy, search for eggs, or gratify the hunting instincts of later life, by stalking parasites and pigments in the field of corpuscles .1 inch, which an oil immersion lens brings to view." His enthusiastic curiosity spread to all medical conditions. He noted the widespread incidence of leprosy and wished that each tribe could have a Leper Reserve in which no hut tax would be collected.

In 1913 he built an operating room: "All our cataract cases have done well: one old lady refuses to go away. She was blind when brought in, now she sees well. Strong spectacles for cataract cases would be a welcome gift." Next year he treated 5 maternity cases in hospital. In 1915 he wrote "the outstanding feature of the year was the epidemic of beri beri, with 10 cases at

Ngara, of which two died. Mr.Dobson the magistrate was killed by a rhinoceros."

The worsening war in Tanganyika, caused the Government to conscript mission doctors in 1917, and Dr.Prentice willingly responded. During the bubonic plague epidemic at Karonga, he telegraphed enthusiastically from New Langenburg that he had found two cases of plague there; "the microscope showed they were short, round ended, various sized, bi-polar staining, bacilli pestis, of bubonic plague."

After the war, he returned to Kasungu to the worsening problems of Sleeping Sickness. By 1924, "the areas devastated by the tsetse fly have increased. Dr.Prentice has called attention to its spread south of Embangweni, round Kasungu, and east to Kota Kota."

His integrity combined with his innate hunting instincts, gave him an enthusiastic medical curiosity. His interest in all disease conditions passed over to his patients, and whole communities became interested in improving health. His life's work is a fine example in Africa today. Health is improved not by philosophies and policies in wordy publications. The personal curiosity of the doctor is the essential guidance needed in every local community. "What are the disease problems in this district? How are they to be solved ?"

After thirty years of devoted Christian service as both priest and doctor in the Livingstonia Mission, Dr.Prentice left Nyasaland with his wife in 1924, to return to Scotland.

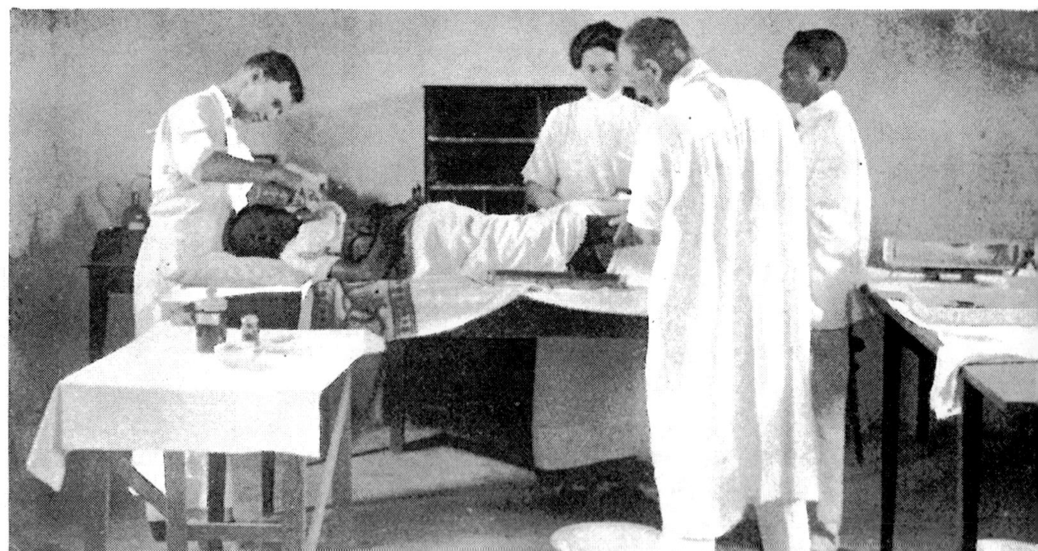

Dr. Prentice operating in Kasungu 1911 with Dr.W.Y.Turner, anaesthetist, Nurse Henderson and Hospital assistant.

19   BACTERIAL DISEASES

The early doctors brought with them perhaps seven useful drugs: quinine, morphia, chloroform, digitalis, local anaesthetics, vaccine lymph, and local antiseptics. Until 1890 only malaria among the infectious diseases had a specific remedy. Treating the others, pneumonia, meningitis, syphilis, etc. meant nursing care; and letting the disease run its course. The outcome depended on the virulence of the disease and the constitution of the patient. There was little the medical attendants could do to influence the outcome. Some of the measures used, blood letting, purging, and sweating, were probably harmful.

In the 1890s, antisera against certain infectious diseases were produced at the Robert Koch Institute in Germany. Dead bacteria, or their toxic by-products, were injected into a horse, and after a few weeks specific proteins (antibodies) were produced against these foreign materials. These could be extracted and concentrated from the horse blood. Antisera were developed against tetanus, typhoid, diphtheria, plague, gas gangrene, and snake venom. Some are still in use today (tetanus and snake venom). They were not always effective, and not without danger from allergic reactions.

Paul Ehrlich at Frankfurt looked for "magic bullets", or chemical guided missiles that would kill bacteria in the body, in the same way as antisera. Various dyes and heavy metal compounds were tried with some success, but the breakthrough came with the 606th compound of Arsenic he tried in 1907. This was useful against syphilis, and was called Salvarsan.

In 1935, Gerard Domagk produced Prontosil from a red dye in Germany. It was very effective against pneumonia, urinary infections, childbirth fever, and meningitis. The active ingredient was a sulphonamide, and modification of this produced a range of life saving drugs, including Dapsone used in leprosy.

In England, Alexander Fleming noticed in 1928 that colonies of staphylococci, a dangerous bacteria, would not grow near a mould that had contaminated a culture plate. The mould was producing a substance that killed bacteria, and he named it Penicillin. At Oxford, Florey and Chain managed to extract and purify penicillin in their laboratory by 1938. It was soon found to be a wonder drug in curing septic infections, and was mass produced by 1943.

Research into other moulds produced a broader range of antibiotics, including Streptomycin and Tetracycline. Later chemical manipulation produced an even greater range of more powerful compounds. Bacteria do develop resistance to some antibiotics. There are unfortunately no similar drugs that are active against viruses except Acyclovir (1977) which is useful in herpes. Much research is being done in this field especially against the Aids virus.

In Malaŵi, even with antibiotics, today infectious diseases account for over 60% of adult admissions to the medical wards and for over half the deaths. The figures for children are similar. In Europe perhaps 10% of admissions would be for infectious diseases, usually pneumonia in elderly patients. The peak age-group in Malaŵi would be 20-30 years.

TETANUS

Wordsworth Poole wrote at Zomba 1895 "one patient was a Makua who shot his foot. He showed signs of tetanus so I took his foot off, but he got worse every hour and died this morning. It is very hard nursing a case of tetanus, every touch brings on spasm." The spasms are produced by a toxin from the bacteria which will only multiply in very damaged tissues although the bacteria and spores are commonly found in the soil.

Dr.Howard in 1910 had not seen many cases of tetanus by the Lake and never in the newborn. The shrivelling umbilical cord gets infected. Newborn tetanus is however seen in Malaŵi today and often is fatal. Antisera can be used in treatment, but it is much better to allow the patient, or mother, to develop their own immunity by injecting the denatured, or safe, toxin before exposure to the disease. Toxoid administration is part of the Extended Programme of Immunization (EPI) for children. Penicillin can only kill the bacteria if there is a good blood supply to the infected area.

DIPHTHERIA

This is another bacterial disease that produces toxins and also obstructs the larynx causing breathing problems. It occurred among some early Europeans. In 1891 Henry Henderson's baby died of it at the Blantyre Mission; Dr.John Bowie also contracted this disease doing a tracheostomy, inserting a tube into the windpipe; and also Mrs. Henderson. Dr.Affleck Scott had seen other European cases. Sporadic cases have been recorded since: 1911 Zomba 4 Africans, and 2 Europeans; 1923 3 cases; 1946 153 cases; 1953 24 cases with 5 deaths. It is very rare today and there are effective antibiotics to treat it.

MENINGITIS

Outbreaks of this often fatal disease affecting the brain have been recorded since the early days. Public health measures including quarantining affected villages,and delaying funeral feasts, could prevent spread. In 1937 there were some hundreds of cases on the Phalombe plain, confined by restricting travel. Dr.Berry, who was in charge, had a small supply of the new sulpha drugs,and he had to deal with other outbreaks the next year.

There was a meningitis outbreak at Fort Johnston and another at Matope where the bridge was being built across the Shire river. There were 700 labourers in crowded quarters. Prontosil was used but the disease was very virulent, some patients dying in 12 hours. The crowded sleeping quarters and the sharing of blankets contributed to the epidemic and when this was corrected, it died out. There were 195 deaths and 362 reported cases.

In 1988 another outbreak of the disease entered Malaŵi, coming to Africa from India and the Middle East. It is especially prevalent in the dry months (July - October) and in young people. It has become a major cause of admission and death, even though effective antibiotics are available

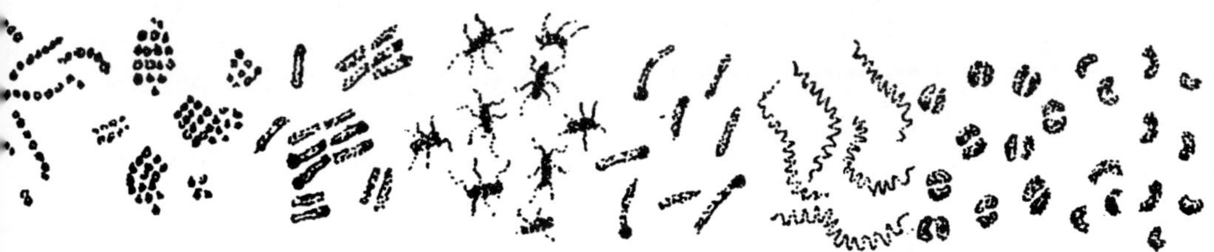

Bacteria causing (L to R) Cellulitis, Abscesses, Diphtheria, Typhoid, Tetanus, Syphillis, Gonorrhoea, Cholera

TYPHOID

This water borne disease is endemic, occurring all the time. It presents as fever with intestinal complications. Dr.Howard believed it was introduced into Blantyre and spread. In 1903 a Typhoid Ward was built and opened at the Blantyre Mission by public subscription.

An official contacted typhoid in Zomba in 1911 and this led to a demand for piped water supplies. In 1924 there were more European cases, and in 1943 it was suggested all should be vaccinated as there was no specific remedy. In 1940, 27 cases with 4 deaths were reported, certainly a gross under-estimate. Today it is common and in spite of effective antibiotics,has a significant mortality. A little over half the population are said to have access to safe water. Improvement of water supplies would decrease the incidence, as it would with the following diseases.

DYSENTERY AND CHOLERA

January 1897 "There has been quite an epidemic of dysentery during the last month in the Shire Highlands and on the River. Mr.Nicoll's (British vice consul) death was due to dysentery."

Diarrhoeal diseases are a significant cause of death especially in malnourished children, the sixth most common cause of death in the under 4 year olds. It is interesting to note that a survey of infant mortality at Karonga in 1932 showed that only 6 out of 101 deaths were thought to be due to diarrhoea. Dr.Austin was surprised at this low figure attributing it to the protection given by prolonged breast feeding.

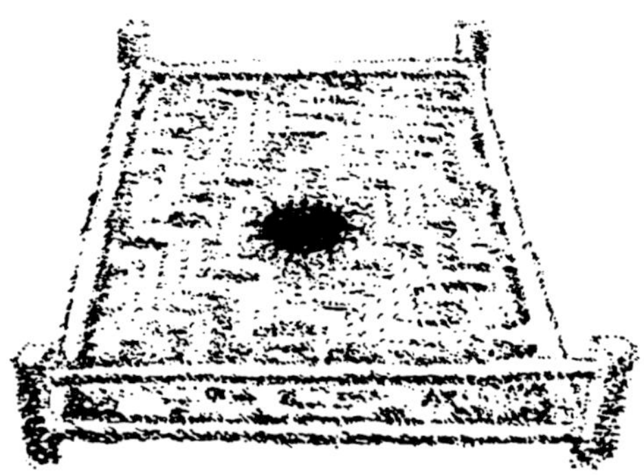

Locally made Cholera bed, Chiradzulu 1990. A bucket is placed below the hole.

Since 1816 successive pandemics of cholera have swept the world from the original one in India. The present pandemic started in 1961 and reached Africa by 1970. It reached Nsanje via Mozambique in September 1973, together with other dysenteries especially shigellosis. By October there had been 282 confirmed cases of cholera, identified by the typical comma shaped bacteria, with 58 deaths. Intensive treatment centres were set up in the hospital, using army tents. 20 - 30 cases a day were admitted and treated. Intravenous fluids were given to counteract severe dehydration and shock due to the pea soup diarrhoea. 23,360 vaccinations were carried out although the value of this is doubted today. Tetracycline was given.

However it spread up to the Shire Highlands, and by the end of 1974 it had been diagnosed throughout Malaŵi. Since then it has been endemic with outbreaks in crowded areas, and near the Lake, Shire River, and Lake Chilwa.

1973 - 1982	
Notified cases of diarrhoea	66,077
Notified cases of cholera	6,253
Deaths - whole group	1,484

Fishermen make straw huts on the floating reeds, 'zimbowela', of Lake Chilwa, and are obviously at risk from this largely water borne disease.

Today, oral rehydration therapy (boiled water

with added sugar and salt) is given for diarrhoeal diseases, with less reliance on antibiotics. Piped water supplies in Malaŵi are safe to drink. Those who only have access to polluted streams and wells are at risk.

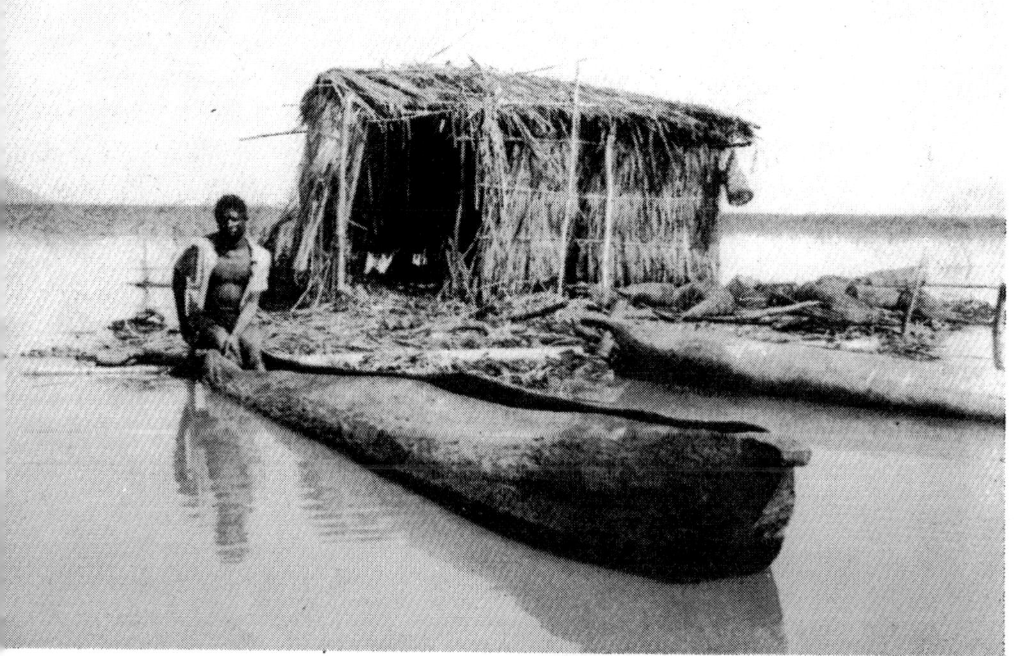

Zimbowela on Lake Chilwa

SEXUALLY TRANSMITTED DISEASES (STD)

These have always been a problem. Dr.Kerr Cross wrote from Karonga in 1896: "Some 200 women were married after the traditional fashion to men of various tribes who had assisted in both the Expeditions (slave wars). I am sorry to report that this has been the means of spreading all forms of impure diseases."

In 1911 there were reports of increase in venereal (STD) disease among Europeans and Africans. The following year the sick rate of Europeans was 13% for malaria and 6% for venereal disease. Salvarsan and Bismuth injections were used for syphilis after the First World War. As often happens, the number of reported cases probably bore only a faint relation to the actual numbers.

In 1935, 1,324 cases were reported and there was a rather impractical ruling that all patients were to be referred to central hospitals for intravenous or muscular injections of Salvarsan. The numbers continued to increase and in 1945 the Colonial Development Fund gave £45,000 over 5 years for treatment. Four years later 22,250 cases were treated free (15,407 syphilis, 6,677 gonorrhoea). By this time sulphonamides were used for gonorrhoea.

Penicillin was used for both in 1951. Gonorrhoea has increasingly become resistant to penicillin, but syphilis luckily has not. Possibly because of this, and the widespread use of penicillin, the actual incidence of syphilis, and its more serious side effects on the brain, may have decreased. Sexually Transmitted Diseases remain among the top ten causes of seeking medical help, and are a major problem in Malaŵi as in the rest of Africa.

YAWS

The terrible skin lesions of this disease were obvious to the early missionaries, especially in the hot wet areas. Dr.Howard in 1900 noticed it was very common along the east shore of the Lake. It is a non-fatal disease caused by a spiral bacillus, similar to the organism causing syphilis, first identified by Castellani in Ceylon in 1905.

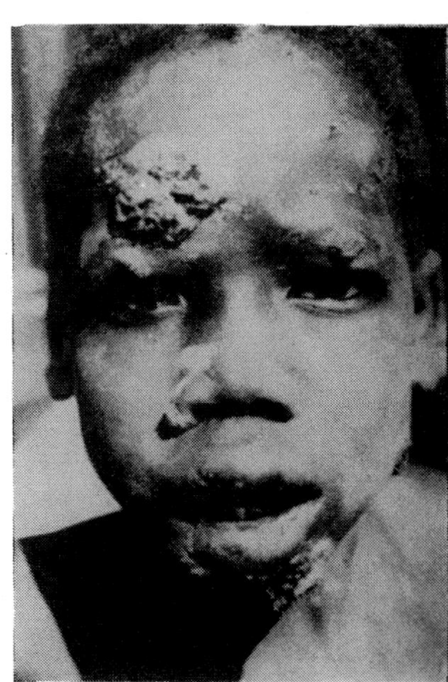

Yaws

In the Dedza district survey by Dr.Davey in 1913, from the typical scars, 16.5% of adults showed evidence of having had the disease. In 1915, 10% of the chronic cases treated in Blantyre were yaws. By 1920 the disease seemed to be on the increase, especially in the Lake villages. 1,776 patients were treated with arsenic or bismuth containing injections. These were quite effective but painful, so many did not complete the three week course. At Likoma patients were asked to pay 5 shillings towards the 6 shilling cost. This was approximately one month's wage, but because the results were so marvellous, friends and relatives would contribute. Occasionally patients would work for it, building or hoeing. In 1949 3,237 cases were reported in the whole country, although no doubt this was an under-estimate. The next year massive eradication campaigns were launched in various parts of the world by WHO using one shot, long acting, penicillin developed a few years before. The results were dramatic. In 1952 4.9% of the population of Karonga were affected but within a few years the disease was eradicated in Malaŵi, although it still occurs in West Africa.

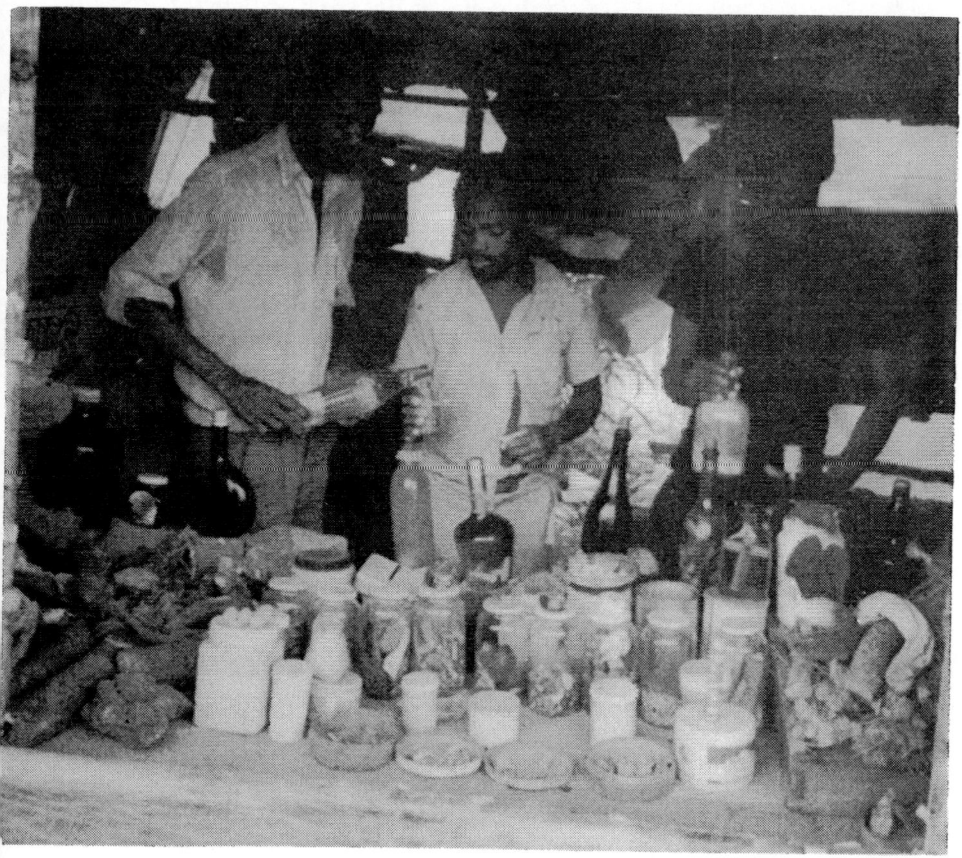

Traditional Medicine Stall. Blantyre 1991. The traditional practitioners generally recognize the value of antibiotics and will often advise patients with infectious diseases to go to a dispensary or hospital.

A family tradition has sustained this medical work for a century. In October 1889, Andrew Murray, from a Scottish Christian family in Cape Province, South Africa, pitched his tent under a fig tree beside the Msungudzi Stream, near the Ngoni Chief Chiwere. He was a priest with a little medical training and had been advised by Dr.Laws to settle there. With Mr.T.C.Vlok, he built a house, laid out fruit and vegetable gardens, and named the place Mvera, it is near modern Salima.

The powerful Chief Chiwere protected these early missionaries in a treacherous situation. Raids by Chief Mpemba were continual, and thousands of slaves were still being transported across the Lake. Witchcraft and the mwabvi poison cup were regular events. Then the Ngoni often sallied forth with shield and assegai to make retaliatory raids against the Chewas and the Yaos, and returned with their faces smeared with white clay if they had been successful.

Andrew Murray opened a dispensary and in the first year 200 people sought help. When he was badly wounded on the scalp by a leopard, he had to stitch his deep cuts himself. Infection developed and he barely survived. Then Mr.Vlok's baby died at birth, and his wife perished from malaria a few days later.

The Chewa Chief Mazengera then asked these missionaries to settle at Nkhoma because his people were harassed by the Ngoni. About 2,000 Chewas were sleeping on the plateau of Nkhoma Mountain at night, with stones ready to hurl at the Ngoni from the High Rock. A Dispensary was started there in 1896.

By 1899, 12,5000 patients were treated in dispensaries and a doctor was needed. Andrew's cousin, Dr.William A.Murray*, who had qualified at Edinburgh, came to Mvera in 1900. He built his house, and then the first Mvera hospital with a grass roof for £80. Here he had to operate on animal wounds, fractures, ulcers, cancer, abdominal problems, and midwifery cases. He trained medical dressers to assist him, and also the first nurse, Sara Lingodzi Nabanda*, who later served the hospital for 34 years. Contemporaries remember Sara's visionary and enlightened sense of commitment to human care. The Nkhoma School of Nursing is named after her.   *Illus. inside covers.

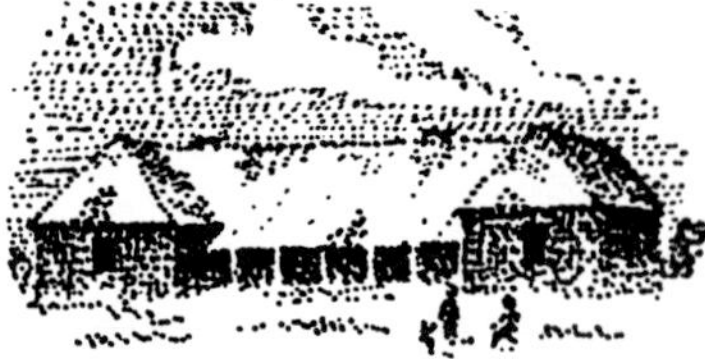

Mvera Hospital 1903.

Dr.Murray visited other dispensaries, often riding one of the white Zanzibari donkeys, which the Mission imported to use for many years before the day of motor cars. One day he received a message at Mlanda, high up in the Dedza Mountains, that a patient was dying at Nkhoma. He sprang into the saddle of his horse 'Hardy' at sunrise, and galloped 80 miles down to the plains to reach Nkhoma before sunset, in time to save a woman's life.

Several more relatives of the Murrays served this Mission. Dr.Pauline* and Dr. William Murray were both born to the wife of a pastor at Mvera in 1902-4. Pauline's parents remembered cutting pieces of biltong for her there: "in the innermost sanctuary of our family life, alone with our small children in the morning or evening, we have indescribably happy experiences; our dear little son is also a jolly little fellow."   *Illus inside front cover

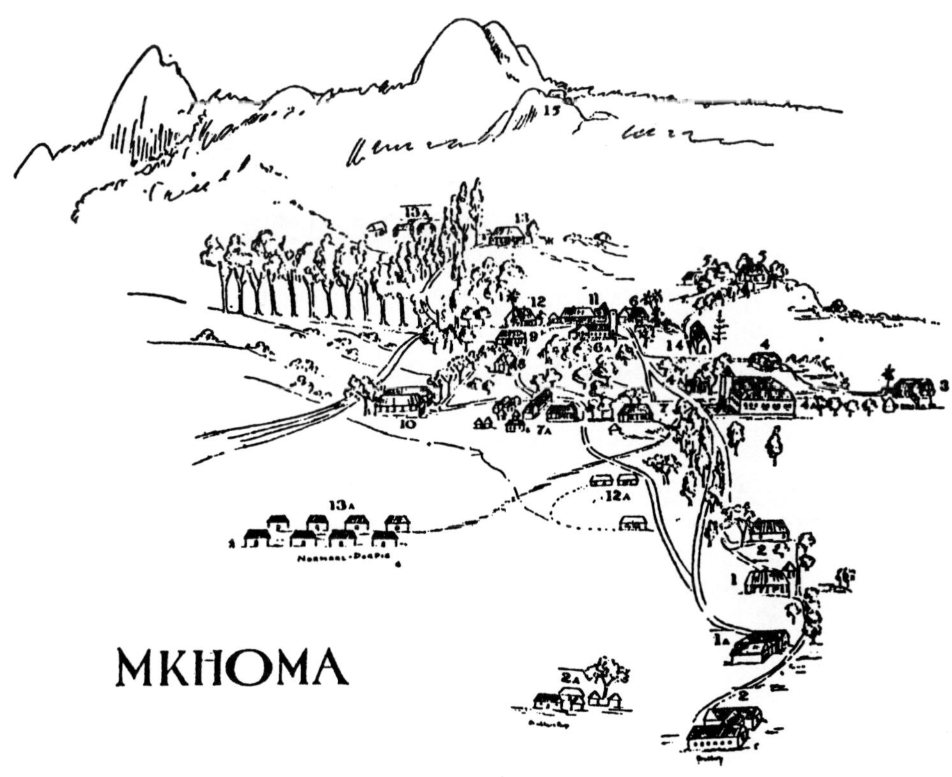

Nkoma (Mkoma is an old spelling) from an early pamphlet. 4A = Head of Mission's house, 6A = Church, 7A = Hospital, 8 = Nurses House, 15 =Rest House on the mountain.

By 1910, tsetse flies and sleeping sickness at Mvera caused the missionaries to move to Nkhoma which at 4,000 feet is very beautiful. The houses are built at different heights on the slopes of the mountain, with fine views from the operating theatre window. From the Peak there is a bird's eye view of Lake Malaŵi to the east and of Zambian mountains to the west.

More stations with dispensaries were opened by the DRC: at Chintembwe, 40 miles north of Mvera, nearly 6,000 feet above sea level, and surrounded by primaeval forest; and at Mchinji in 1914 "this was right in the heart of lion country, many people have been attacked or killed by lions there." The outbreak of war in 1914 caused the Government to construct many roads in this area. Carts drawn by a span of oxen became a familiar sight. The mission medical work progressed steadily, by 1916 there were 9 outlying health units. Supplies were short and wounds might be dressed with local kapok or tree cotton which was teased out, boiled, and dried in the oven. *Castor Oil Plant* Raw castor oil, and banana leaves were also used, the latter being practical for maternity cases.

By 1924, more than 75,000 patients were treated in the DRC hospitals, a third of them with ulcers, and burns cases, accidents, maternity patients, and cases of yaws, syphilis, scabies, and ringworm, were common.

Several more medical Murrays arrived, including Dr.Jeannette Murray, the first lady doctor, in 1925, Dr.L.Murray (1923-7), Dr.J.F.L.Murray (1925-36), and Dr.Pauline Murray who pioneered midwifery teaching at Mlanda hospital. When Pauline married Mr.Praetorius, he was ill with malaria, so she walked beside the machila which carried him up to the Rest House on Nkhoma Mountain for their honeymoon.

In 1929, the Mission started an isolation camp for lepers at Katete Stream near Madetsa. Special units for tuberculosis and maternity patients were started in the hospital in the '30s. Dr.Renaldo Retief, a relative of the Murrays, started specialized ophthalmology at Nkhoma in 1928, concentrating on cataract surgery. The eye unit was opened in 1955, and for thirty years Dr.C.Blignaut has continued the ophthalmological services offered by this Mission, which has gained an international reputation.

The picturesque Dutch tiled roofs, the sturdy gardens, the passing cart drawn by a span of oxen, and the devoted family atmosphere of successive generations of South African doctors, still enhance Nkhoma Mission Hospital.

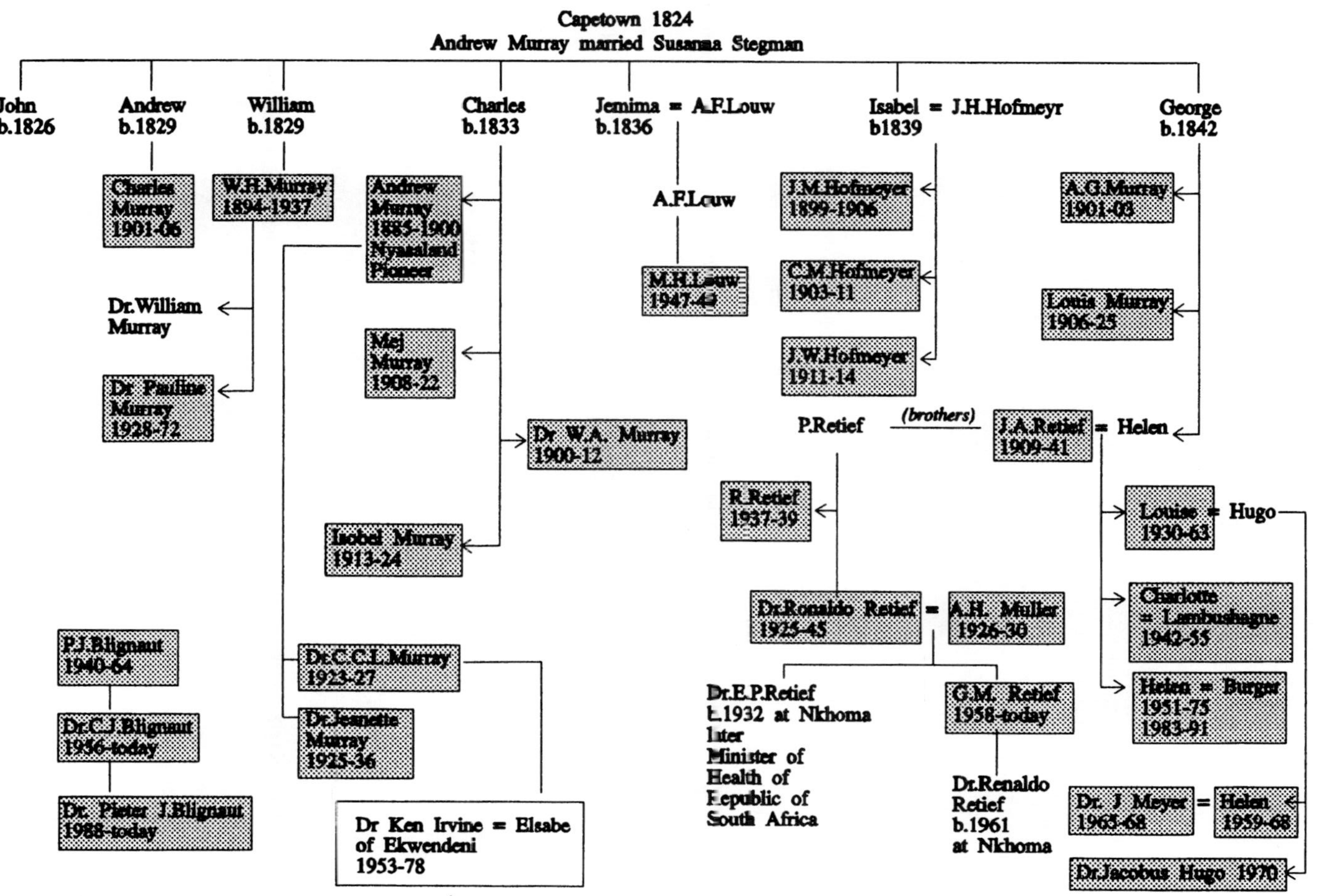

Capetown 1824
Andrew Murray married Susanna Stegman
John b.1826
Andrew b.1829
William b.1829
Charles b.1833
Jemima = A.F.Louw b.1836
Isabel = J.H.Hofmeyr b.1839
George b.1842
Charles Murray 1901-06
W.H.Murray 1894-1937
Andrew Murray 1885-1900 Nyasaland Pioneer
A.F.Louw
J.M.Hofmeyr 1899-1906
A.G.Murray 1901-03
Dr.William Murray
M.H.Louw 1947-49
C.M.Hofmeyr 1903-11
Louisa Murray 1906-25
Dr Pauline Murray 1928-72
Mej Murray 1908-22
J.W.Hofmeyr 1911-14
Dr W.A. Murray 1900-12
P.Retief
(brothers)
J.A.Retief 1909-41 = Helen
R.Retief 1937-39
Louise = Hugo 1930-63
Isobel Murray 1913-24
Dr.Ronaldo Retief 1925-45 = A.H. Muller 1926-30
Charlotte = Lambashagne 1942-55
P.J.Blignaut 1940-64
Dr.C.C.L.Murray 1923-27
Dr.E.P.Retief b.1932 at Nkhoma later Minister of Health of Republic of South Africa
G.M. Retief 1958-today
Helen = Burger 1951-75 1983-91
Dr.C.J.Blignaut 1956-today
Dr.Jeanette Murray 1925-36
Dr.Renaldo Retief b.1961 at Nkhoma
Dr. J Meyer 1963-68 = Helen 1959-68
Dr. Pieter J.Blignaut 1988-today
Dr Ken Irvine = Elsabe of Ekwendeni 1953-78
Dr.Jacobus Hugo 1970
Dates in shaded boxes indicate service in Malaŵi D.R.C.

21 MEDICAL TRAINING

"Ars longa, vita brevis" Hippocrates 400 BC

"The life so short, the craft so long to learn"

As soon as hospitals were built, it became possible to teach local staff. However, training was limited by previous levels of education. Until 1940, there were no secondary schools in Nyasaland. Uneducated apprentices could only be taught some routine practical procedures as Medical Orderlies. Literate and numerate candidates could understand some simple concepts of disease and treatment, and be trained as Medical Dressers. Students with full primary school education were later given a more scientific education as Hospital Assistants.

Blantyre Mission Hospital trained the first Medical Dressers in Nyasaland as soon as it was built in 1896. Dr.Neil MacVicar arrived and foresaw that Blantyre Hospital would become the great teaching hospital for the country, with smaller hospitals dependent on it.

John Gray Kufa was the first person to receive formal Medical Assistant training in Nyasaland. His career was remarkable. He left his home at the Kongone mouth of the Zambesi, to join the Blantyre missionaries in 1885. He was one of the first seven deacons ordained in Blantyre Church in 1892, and five years later he married Dorothy Ndana there. In August 1898 the Mission reported : "John Gray Kufa has passed with distinction (90%) an examination upon the course of minor medicine and surgery prescribed for hospital dressers. He is the first of the hospital assistants who has attempted this examination, and we heartily congratulate him on his success. It is the result of diligent study, together with careful attention to practical details of the work. When, the week after the examination, John Gray left for Anguruland, he took with him a large supply of medicines and dressings. He is to have charge of a Station and Dispensary there." The Angurus were a clan of the Lomwe tribe who were then moving into the Thyolo area. Tragically, John Gray Kufa was executed in January 1915 for associating with John Chilembwe's rebellion against the British at Chiradzulu. After this rebellion the government viewed the Missions with suspicion.

David Mothela from Domasi passed the same qualifying examination at Blantyre Hospital a year later, and returned home to take charge of a dispensary.

A few interesting notes survive about these pioneer local medical staff:

In 1903 "Che Samuel at Chiradzulu does simple medical work confined almost entirely to the dressing of ulcers and toes rotting off with jiggers. Because children howl if their mothers try to pick the fleas out, they let the children's feet get into a horrible state."

At Panthumbi dispensary among the Ngonis, near Ntcheu, Che Harry Kambwiri was in charge in 1903: "People with ulcers are constantly waiting about to have their sores dressed. Others come with cuts and burns which Harry can dress and bandage."It was perhaps a tribute to Harry Kambwiri that "eight Panthumbi boys are learning at Blantyre Mission Hospital".

In the North, Dr.Innes was keenly interested in teaching: "In landing at Bandawe Mission in 1899, I was impressed with the potential value of local assistants in medical work...patients respond wonderfully to treatment by their own people."

Dr.Boxer at Bandawe noted in 1902: "My Dispensary Assistant is of very great use to me now. He has been trained in the elements of pharmacy and can mix prescriptions. All the ulcer cases are in his hands, and I leave chloroform entirely in his charge."

At Blantyre Mission, Dr.Caverill proposed a more systematic training of medical staff in 1904:

1) Dressers would be trained for six months, boys would learn the art of dressing wounds and giving out stock medicines.

2) Hospital Attendants would have a three year training with examinations and a certificate.

3) Hospital Assistants would do further specialized training after the basic three year course, and would be able to take an important place in the central hospital.

In 1909, The Colonial Government at last officially recognized the Training Course for Hospital Assistants, who had first passed Standard 3 at school. The first Hospital Assistant trained at Livingstonia Mission at Khondowe graduated in 1909: "Daniel Gondwe, who was trained at this Institution has been very useful in this work, and is becoming deservedly popular among the people", and four years later at Ekwendeni it was noted "Daniel Gondwe has the confidence of the people, and at the Dispensary and in the homes of patients relieves much suffering."

Dr.Innes, after ten years at Karonga Mission, was asked to share with Dr.Laws the burden of teaching at David Gordon Memorial Hospital, when it opened in 1911. "There are two students at present, one for the course of hospital orderly, and one for the higher grade of hospital assistant."

At Blantyre, Dr.MacFarlane came to organize a four year training course, with an extra year of practical work afterwards in 1914. In the same year Dr.Laws formally objected to the Government putting under-qualified persons on the Medical Register. He also asked for a national register of trained Medical Assistants, Nurses, and Midwives, and asked the Government to set national qualifying examinations.

The Great War created an immediate demand for more medical staff and Dr. MacVicar responded with an interesting scheme in Blantyre to train uneducated boys as hospital apprentices. The students learned English and were given practical training. Many Ngoni boys applied for this course and a few girls also completed it.

The first local nurse in Nyasaland received a touching tribute when she died at Livingstonia Hospital in 1915: Maria Chilimbirano had been captured as a slave, later coming to Livingstonia in 1901. She was the senior African nurse, and died of heart failure: "The human motherly touch of Maria must be a life memory to many; no one would say she was clever; her concern was of the right sort, seeking the spiritual as well as the physical welfare of her patients. Can it be wrong to say we grudge her going? We miss her greatly. She was ready to do extra work for the sick, and sat up with an ill woman at night after her day's work was done, with never a grumble." In 1909 the Dutch Reformed Mission began the training of nurses at Mvera. Mrs. Sara Nabanda, the first nurse, served the Mission for 34 years.

The Universities Mission started systematic Medical Dresser training on Likoma Island in 1912, and gradually teaching was extended to women. Nkhota Kota Hospital reported in 1915 "In the womens' ward I am training a woman to help and she has proved skilful in doing the dressings. She earned great credit from the Government doctor when he brought in an accident case. At Mvera they have a woman to dress the female patients, and Fanny at Bandawe Hospital is a wonderfully useful person".

In 1917, five boys and one girl received their Hospital Assistant Certificates at Blantyre "remarkable advances have been made in training African staff both male and female: ten years ago they were uneducated, now we have a fully organized system of apprenticeship with schoolboys who have passed fourth standard, being indentured to us for five years. The high standard of their work and study has impressed many."

Other more basic levels proliferated: 25 Dawa Boys (Yao for medicine) were trained at Likoma Island Mission in 1919. "The boys start at 15 years; they begin to use a microscope under supervision and are very keen about examining specimens for bilharzia, hookworm etc. Over 1,000 examinations were made by them in one hospital in six months. They are also taught some medicine and surgery. They prepare the theatre, and visit the villages."

By 1930, the Universities Mission noted that one of these dispensary assistants "had 25,000 outpatients attendances in one year and visited many sick in neighbouring villages. He sends patients up to Likoma Hospital. He has his small microscope: recently he saved a priest from relapses of tick fever by taking blood slides at the right time and sending them to the doctor at Likoma."

A more advanced Medical Assistant College was established by Dr. Laws at Livingstonia. In 1924, "during the months the hospital was without a nurse, the Medical Assistants rose gloriously to the occasion and worked well. The medical classes for our students have continued throughout the year, the subjects being Biology, Physiology, Anatomy, and clinical material. On many occasions we felt the need for an X-Ray plant." Proper courses for training nurses were begun at Kondowe, Mvera, Mlanda, and Nkhoma hospitals in 1925.

The following year saw the return to Nyasaland of the first local doctor, Dr.Daniel S. Malekebu. He had studied medicine at Meharry Medical School, in Nashville, Tennessee, U.S.A. It was a leading Negro Medical College. After qualifying as a doctor there, Dr.Malekebu came home to re-open Providence Industrial Mission at Chiradzulu.

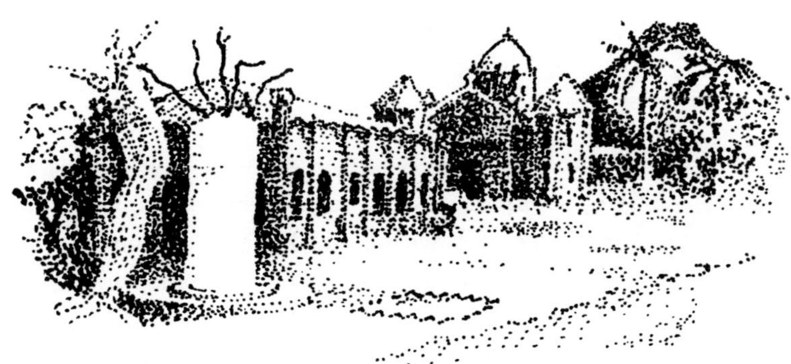

Providence Industrial Mision today. The white concrete pillar encloses a tree trunk. The inscription reads:- "Under this tree Dr. & Mrs. Malekebu re-opened P.I.M. 8 June 1926 as a church."

The official Sanderson Report of 1926 to the Chief Medical Officer stated "the extension of the Health Services is entirely dependent on the formation of a local staff. A single handed doctor can do little." Also in 1926, the General Medical Council of Nyasaland was set up to examine and register staff. Official recognition was extended to Livingstonia's training of Medical and Hospital Assistants and Nurses.

There were still staff shortages. In 1930 Nurse Simpkin reported from Likoma Island "We very much hope to begin systematic training of young women. At present the hospital cook is able to lend a hand, she is capable of looking after patients as they come round after anaesthetic."

The Government reported in 1934 "the rural dispensary scheme, through lack of supervision, is in a somewhat stagnant state.... there is a great need to train Africans in methods of disease prevention, village hygiene, better house construction, and sanitary education." Blantyre Mission maintained a high standard of teaching and received an annual government grant for this. The first Government Medical Training School was opened at Zomba in 1936, with courses for medical dressers, nurses and midwives, laboratory assistants, and sanitary inspectors.

<table>
<tr><td colspan="3" align="center">Government Medical Establishment</td></tr>
<tr><td>Year</td><td>Hospital Assistants</td><td>Medical Dressers</td></tr>
<tr><td>1927</td><td>3</td><td>130</td></tr>
<tr><td>1929</td><td>5</td><td>145</td></tr>
<tr><td>1931</td><td>18</td><td>166</td></tr>
<tr><td>1933</td><td>18</td><td>182</td></tr>
<tr><td>1935</td><td>12</td><td>182</td></tr>
<tr><td>1937</td><td>16</td><td>201</td></tr>
<tr><td>1939</td><td>32</td><td>215</td></tr>
</table>

1935 Five junior Hospital Assistants
Mr. T.H.K. Chirwa, MrJ.B.Wachepa, Mr.G.Ndovi, Mr.G.Nyirenda, Mr.R.C.Undi.

THE SECOND WORLD WAR

In 1939, nine out of eighteen Government doctors in Nyasaland were transferred to the army, together with their Medical Dressers. There was an immediate demand for more army dressers, so the Government trained them as quickly as possible. A class of 25 was visualized at Zomba Hospital with six months training. However, there was so much local enthusiasm for this course that "we found 43 had been signed on for the first course in 1940 - the first class of trained recruits should be ready to go North by June 1941."

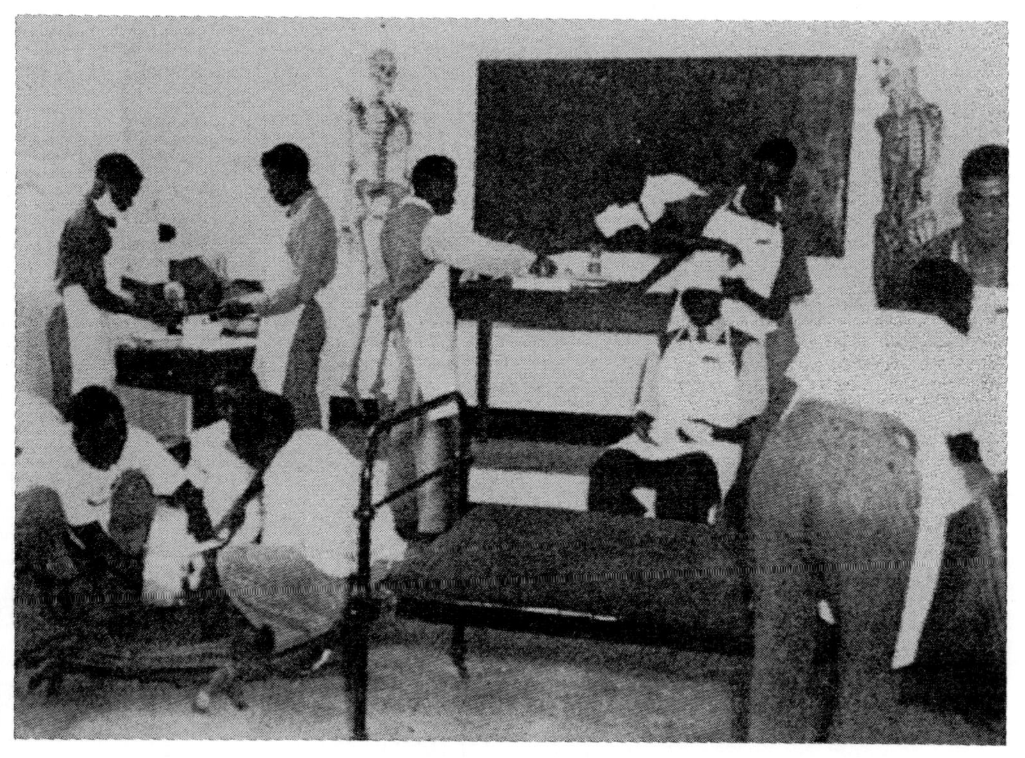

Medical Aide Training School 1951.

Hospital Assistants now had to do the work of doctors: "the maintenance of medical services depended largely on our African Hospital Assistants, who, if properly trained, are capable of excellent work with little supervision. They have been in charge of the following District Hospitals this year (1940): Chiradzulu, Chikwawa, Upper Shire, Ntcheu, Dedza, Dowa, Kasungu, and Nkhata Bay. One Hospital Assistant who has been given some surgical training at Zomba, is proving a competent and successful surgeon." Zomba Training School expanded. In 1942 the first Surgical Specialist in Nyasaland, Mr.M.A.W. Roberts F.R.C.S. was posted at Zomba Hospital and started proper surgical teaching to the third year Hospital Assistants.

Improvements in secondary school education in Nyasaland made possible more advanced paramedical training in the post-war years. Zomba Training school was upgraded. By 1947 there were 25 students in the course, and a new two year basic course for Hospital Assistants was started, to be followed by a third year of specialized training in surgery, medicine, anaesthetics, etc. Medical Dressers were still the mainstay of the rural health services in 1949: "A great deal of work is required to be done to overtake the tremendous backlog of maintenance necessary at Rural Dispensaries. Hospital Aides, travelling on their own bicycles, carry a small stock of drugs with them and visit villages within 10 miles of their Dispensary". However "shortage of Medical Aides continues to be acute, and the rural dispensary service has been maintained with difficulty."

THE FEDERATION OF RHODESIA AND NYASALAND 1952-63

The greatly increased health budget available during this decade made possible an expansion of training by Government: "in Nyasaland, Medical Aides, Health, Midwifery, and Nursing Assistants, are trained to a Ministry of Health standard. Selected Medical Aides can undergo two further years of training and qualify as Medical Assistants."

By 1961 "Medical and Laboratory Assistants and Midwives are trained at Blantyre, Medical Aides at Lilongwe, Health Assistants and Assistant Nurses at Zomba." Details of advances in training of nurses and medical assistants since 1963 are given in the chapter on independent Malaŵi.

Almost a century after John Gray Kufa began his medical career at the Blantyre Mission, the new Medical College has opened in Blantyre with 14 medical students who have received their initial training in Britain. They come home to work in a well established service of trained personnel. The many grades and specializations of Malaŵi's Medical Assistants and Clinical Officers has always been the backbone of the nation's medical service. Many other African countries have been glad to employ them, and could with advantage copy the Malaŵian system of training.

These Medical Assistants and Clinical Officers have been enterprising in taking medical care to all rural areas, often making difficult journeys on foot, by bicycle, or by boat. With their extra specialized training in medicine, surgery, ophthalmology, leprosy, dentistry, TB, pharmacy, obstetric surgery, AIDS, anaesthetics, radiology, and orthopaedics, they have been able to offer competent care to many categories of sick people. More slowly, nurses and midwives have been trained and are much needed for maternal and child health services.

The new young Malaŵian doctors will bring an active scientific curiosity to diagnose and perceive the causes of medical and surgical conditions. This is greatly needed if the whole community is to participate with them in solving some of the disease problems of the country.

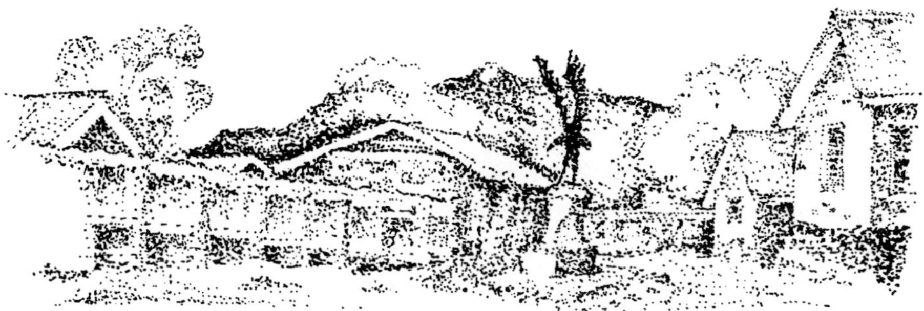

1991 Teaching Annex for Medical College at Queen Elizabeth Hospital. Soche Mountain behind. The cast iron eagle is a memorial to Dr.R.Laws the first medical teacher.

Nguludi Mission today. These old buildings are just above the Hospital where there is a Nurses Training School. Near by there is a Training School for Teachers of the Deaf and a Blind School.(See p.150).

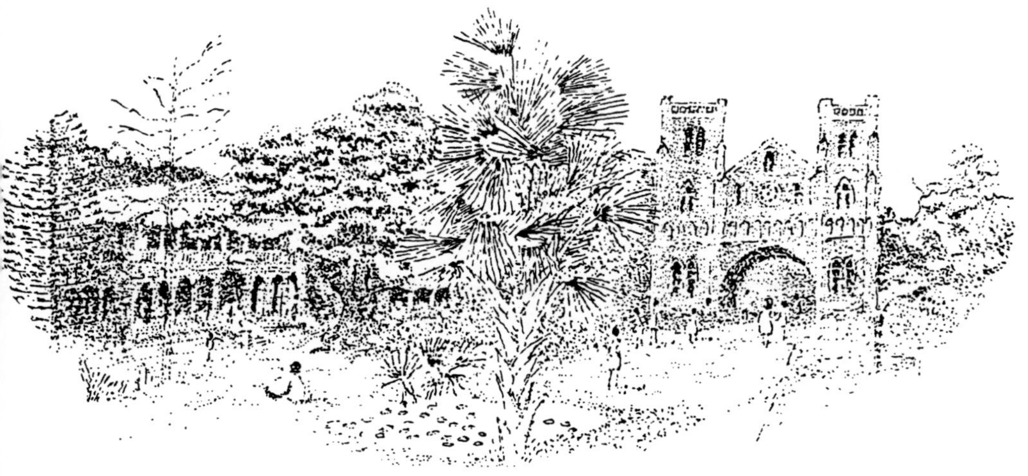

22 TUMOURS

The early doctors were kept busy dealing with trauma, infectious disease, and sanitary measures. "Cancer is not very common" was a comment by Dr.Kerr Cross in 1898, after working for ten years in the Karonga area. In 1925, the Protectorate Annual Health Report mentions only 13 skin tumours in Blantyre and Zomba. There was a general feeling among health workers that malignant disease was rare in Africa. Even in those early days, this was almost certainly wrong. Patients were maybe unwilling to come for treatment for a disease they suspected to be incurable.

The health services could not confirm a diagnosis by microscopical examinations of tissue until 1928. The average life expectancy in the 1920s in much of Africa was probably 30 years, so there would have been few older people around, and cancer tends to be associated with old age. Before the 1950s much was known about parasitic and infectious disease, but it was only with the opening of Medical Schools in Africa that facilities improved, and the full extent of the problem became known.

BURKITT'S LYMPHOMA

Dr.Dennis Burkitt came to Nyasaland in an old Ford estate car in 1961 from the prestigious Makere Medical School at Kampala, Uganda. He was on his famous tumour safari, and visited 56 hospitals in East and Central African countries, travelling 10,000 miles in 10 weeks. The founder of Kampala hospital, Sir Albert Cook, had noted that tumours of the jaw were common in children. These tumours were not seen in Europe or South Africa.

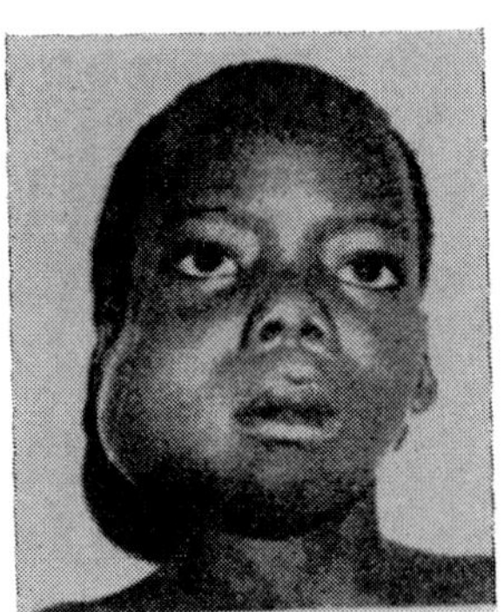

Burkitt's Lymphoma before and after treatment

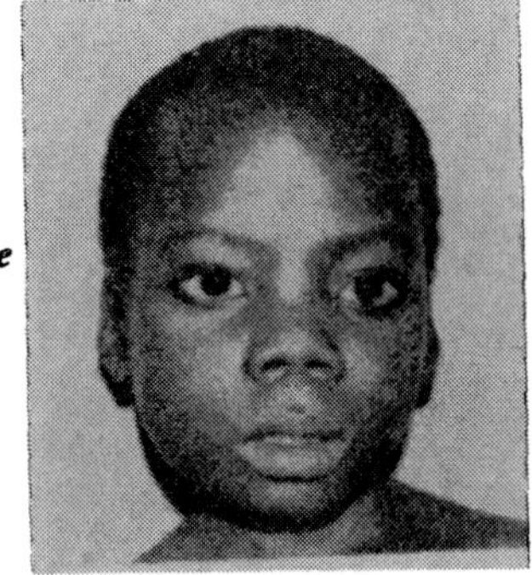

Burkitt decided to map out the distribution of this tumour that usually killed within months. In the course of this safari, he found that where the average temperature fell below 60°F., the tumour did not occur. Thus in Malaŵi it is not found above 3,000 feet, [1,000 feet in Swaziland, 5,000 feet in Tanzania]. In 1989, there were 60 children in Malaŵi diagnosed as Burkitt's Lymphoma, which is now the name of the tumour. As well as the jaws, it can affect many other sites, the abdomen especially. It comprises about 30% of all tumours in children.

In 1964 a new herpes virus, 'Epstein Barr', was isolated from a tissue culture of one of these tumours. Later it was found that all African children with the tumour had antibodies to the virus (i.e. evidence of infection). However the virus is widespread in the community. It is believed that it is the infection by EB virus early in a child's life, and the prevalence of malaria, that together are factors causing the tumour. Malarial mosquitoes are not common where the temperature falls below 60° F.

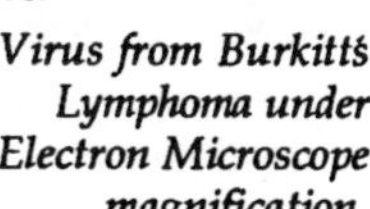

Virus from Burkitts Lymphoma under Electron Microscope magnification.

Burkitt knew that surgery was of no value in the treatment. The tumours are often multiple and grow very fast. Radiotherapy might have been expected to help, but there were and are no facilities in Kampala for this. He was, however, able to obtain cytotoxic drugs from an American source. These drugs kill rapidly dividing cells such as occur in some cancers. He and the patients were gratified to see the tumours melting away over a few days, and sometimes never growing again, so the children could be labelled cured.

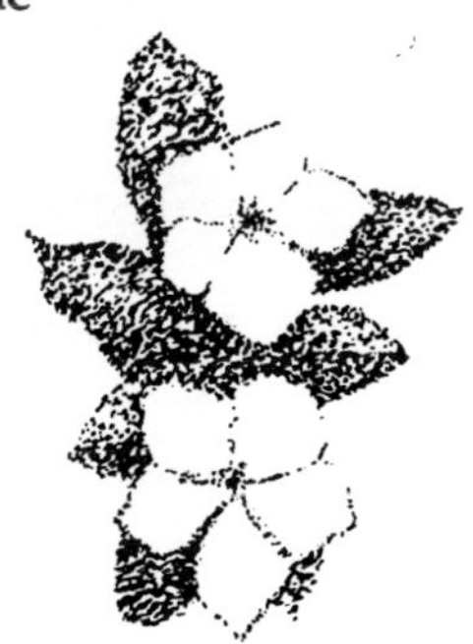

One of the cytotoxic drugs is called Vincristine, which is extracted from the Vinca species, a very common flower growing around Malaŵian village houses.

Vinca.

KAPOSI'S SARCOMA

This is another malignant disease, and is becoming much more common. It also sometimes responds well to cytotoxic drugs. In 1872 in Vienna, Moricz Kaposi described 5 patients with "multiple vascular sarcomas of the skin, bluish nodules." It was later found to be more common among Jews in the U.S.A., but there was no difference in prevalence between the whites and blacks there. It was however a rare disease, only 0·02% of all malignancies in the U.S.A.

In 1934 there were cases described in Nigeria and by 1960 it became obvious that it was in fact quite a common disease in Africa.

Recently a change in the disease has occurred and the numbers are rapidly increasing. In 1989 there were 188 cases confirmed by biopsy. A much more aggressive form of the disease is seen affecting different areas of the body. This was noted first in Zambia in 1983, and when the facilities for laboratory investigation were available, it was shown that these patients were Aids sufferers. It is seen so frequently today, many new cases each week so that it is well recognized by health workers and biopsies are rarely necessary.

Burkitt's Lymphoma is almost never seen in affluent societies, and Kaposi's Sarcoma is rare. There are other malignant diseases common here and rare in the West, and vice versa as can be seen below.

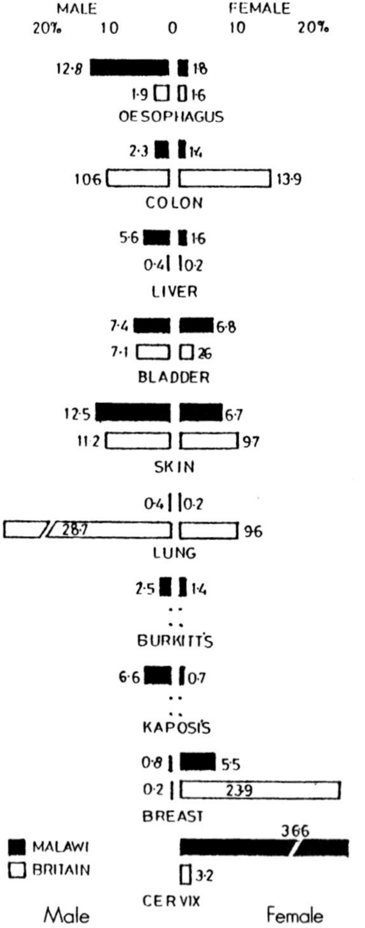

Kaposi's Sarcoma in Malaŵi 1967-85, before Aids Related Kaposi's Sarcoma appeared

Average 28 new cases each year all over the country.
Male:Female 13:1   7% of all biopsied tumours
Mainly affects the legs and is slow growing

SELECTED CANCERS - as a percentage of all body sites

Site	MALAŴI		BRITAIN	
	M	F	M	F
Oesophagus	12·8	1·8	1·9	1·6
Colon/rectum	2·3	1·4	10·6	13·9
Liver	5·6	1·6	0·4	0·2
Bladder	7·4	6·8	7·1	2·6
Skin	12·5	6·7	11·2	9.7
Breast	0·8	5·5	0·2	23·9
Cervix	-	36·6	-	3·2
Lung	0·4	0·2	28·7	9·6
Burkitt's lymphoma	2·5	1·4	<0·01	<0·01
Kaposi's sarcoma*	6·6	0·7	<0·01	<0·01

*Since 1985 the figures for Malaŵi for KS have greatly increased and it is now probably the most common tumour(Aids related).

It is very obvious that there are great differences in the incidence of certain tumours. We have an idea why this is so in some cases.

LIVER CANCER

The difference is not simply racial, it is not common among the black population of U.S.A. or U.K. Several factors are thought to contribute to the high incidence in Malaŵi, and in Africa generally. It is probably among the four commonest tumours in men in rural areas. The virus hepatitis B is over 10 times more common in the Malaŵian population than in that of the U.K. It causes infectious hepatitis or jaundice but it may be a co-factor in the cause of liver cancer. Cirrhosis of the liver is also common, due to malnutrition, alchohol, and infections; and cirrhotic livers are more likely to develop cancer than normal ones.

A possible chemical cause of liver cancer came to light in a curious way in 1961. In that year in the U.K. thousands of turkeys were dying of liver failure. After considerable investigation it seemed as though the common factor in their deaths was that they had eaten feed made from groundnuts. This batch of groundnuts had the common mould, aspergillus flavus, contaminating it. Later, other sources of groundnuts were linked to animal deaths in other parts of the world. A highly toxic substance known as 'aflatoxin' could be extracted from these mouldy groundnuts. Animal experiments showed that in high doses it killed, causing liver failure; however in very small doses over many months it acted as a cancer agent or 'carcinogen' causing the development of tumours in rat livers. Groundnuts are a very nutritious source of protein but it is possible that when contaminated and mouldy, they play a part in the production of liver, and maybe, other cancers in man.

LUNG CANCER

Perhaps the best known group of carcinogens are contained in tobacco tar. The difference in the incidence of lung (bronchus) cancer between Britain, (where it is a prime cause of cancer death), and Malaŵi can be explained by smoking habits. Malaŵians are not heavy smokers although tobacco is their main export! Increasing numbers of young men however are now taking up this habit.

BLADDER CANCER

Bladder cancer may be related to a carcinogen. The type of cancer in Britain, called transitional cell cancer, is known to be linked to smoking and sometimes to chemicals used in the dye industry. The Malaŵian type of cancer, squamous cell carcinoma, is different. It may be difficult to diagnose in its early stages since some symptoms are similar to bilharzia. Certainly there is a relationship between bilharzia and bladder carcinoma. It is thought that bilharzia causes victims to suffer from chronic bacterial bladder infections. The bacteria produce a chemical carcinogen, nitrosamine, and it is this that over the years causes a gradual malignant change to occur in the bladder lining.

OESOPHAGEAL CANCER

The figures for oesophageal cancer show how much more common it is among Malaŵian males than U.K. males. Patients arrive in a late stage at the hospitals, unable to swallow food because the tumour is obstructing the gullet. There are ten times more men than women. In other areas of the world where the disease is common, there are relatively more women. In South Africa the sex ratio is M2:F1, and this increase in the number of women has occurred during the past 20 years. From South African records, it seems as though the disease in both sexes is a recent phenomenon, starting 40 years ago, and spreading north. Even today it is much more common in East Africa than West Africa. These differences are puzzling, possibly explained in part by carcinogens in locally brewed beer and spirits.

CANCER OF THE BREAST AND CERVIX (NECK OF THE WOMB)

The greatest difference between Malaŵi and the Westernized countries is seen in these two cancers of women. They are related to differences in child bearing and rearing. Cervical cancer is associated with early childbearing and multiple pregnancies. The average number of children per mother in Malaŵi is 7·6, in Britain it is less than 2. This suggests that there may a sexually transmitted agent, possibly a combination of a herpes and a papilloma (wart) virus. Evidence for this is found in most cases of the disease.

Cancer of the cervix is not seen in virgin women, but breast cancer may be.
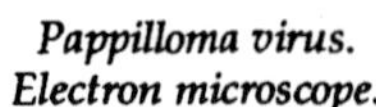
Early pregnancy and breast feeding seems to protect women from breast cancer. Other known factors are dietary and familial. It is certainly the most important cancer in European women, and it seems to be becoming more common among urban Africans, probably due to some of the factors discussed above.

Pappilloma virus.
Electron microscope.

DIET AND CANCER

Dietary factors probably explain the great differences in many diseases. The high animal fat, low fibre, diet of Western countries may lead to a higher incidence of diseases of affluence. These include appendicitis, diverticulitis, gall bladder disease, diabetes, coronary heart disease, and cancer of the breast, lung, colon, and rectum. This was a subject Burkitt turned to after leaving Kampala. Some groups in the West who are vegetarian, and do not smoke or drink alchohol, have a much lower incidence of these diseases than their compatriots. Africans and Asians who live in the West for years eating western food, tend to get these diseases.

SKIN CANCER

This has some topical interest, with the fears of the loss of the ozone layer in the atmosphere, due to certain gases used in refrigerators and aerosols. The ozone layer filters out some ultra-violet rays from the sun. U-V rays can cause sunburn in whites and in albino negroes. Black people are protected by their pigment from sunburn. White people and albinos may get chronic sunburn on exposed areas of their faces and hands, and this may lead to gradual malignant change, and the development of skin cancer. If treated early, these cancers can be completely cured, but unfortunately many albinos come late with advanced multiple tumours. It is very important that they have adequate protection with hats and long sleeved clothes.

How is it that skin cancer is so common in Malaŵi, for it is not only seen in albinos? It is usually due to malignant changes occurring in chronic tropical ulcers. Tropical ulcers were noted in the early days by the missionaries. Indeed the most common task for the early medical assistants was to dress these ulcers. In 1925, there were 369 admissions, out of a total of 3,539, for skin ulcers in Blantyre and Zomba African hospitals. They are still common today. They occur on the lower leg and are probably due to a combination of chronic irritation, malnutrition, and poor hygiene. They remain difficult to cure. Over the years, the cycle of breakdown and healing at the edge of the ulcer leads to malignant change. The now cancerous ulcer may erode the shin bone and require amputation to cure it.

It can be seen from the selection above that there is enough known about the factors involved in some cancers to allow attempts at prevention. Public health measures and better health education could reduce the incidence of some tumours and might enable the sufferers to come for treatment early in the disease, when a cure might be possible.

23   THE CATHOLIC MISSIONS

In December 1889, four White Fathers, led by Fr.Lechaptois of France reached Mponda's village at Mangochi. The powerful Yao Chief Mponda II was busy looting, burning, and kidnapping slaves, in villages around. The Fathers, in their sandals and white habits, tended the sick for 18 months and then left because of the slave war. They saw the tragedy of polygamy and slavery: "15 January 1890 Gunfire during the night. Mponda murdering one of his wives. The corpse was thrown in the river and her effects burned.
3 October 1890 This afternoon one of Mponda's wives suffering from some nervous complaint, tried to drown herself close by. We went out to fetch her in a boat and pulled her in to the bank. Then we took her to her noble spouse who had her well and truly garrotted. He took the same precautions with another of his wives who was suffering from the same complaint."
13 October 1890 "one of the slave traders visits us... one look at his face, though his gaze will not meet yours, is to feel a shiver of fear run through your body."
In 1901 the Montfort Fathers started the first Catholic Mission at Nzama near Ntcheu. Then the Nursing Sisters of La Sagesse arrived. Travelling in machilas, their safari caravan set out from Blantyre in 1904 to camp in villages along the Shire River and then to climb 5,000 feet up the steep Kirk Mountains. They arrived to the singing and dancing of the Ngoni people, and sang a celebration Magnificat with the Fathers. Lunch was of venison brought back from the hunt by Fr.Deau. The Sisters visited the Ngoni Chief Njobulema whose many wives were seated outside their houses.

SISTER JACQUES

Nurse/Sr.Jacques du Saveur from France came to take charge of this Mission in 1909 "where she won all hearts, an excellent administrator....she made Nzama into a little paradise." Then she moved to the new Mission at Utale where damp marshy land and the torrid heat of the plain threatened the new station. "With her bright and winning way, she helped others...she had the gift of sweetening even the most bitter medicine."

Soon the dark clouds of World War I shrouded life.The British Governor appealed for nurses to join the army to care for African soldiers. "To my great satisfaction I am to take part in this expedition. We are preparing linen and cooking equipment, the Fathers have made folding chairs and a table....we will go by lorry from Limbe to Fort Johnston, where a boat will take us up the Lake to Karonga Military Camp."

August 1st 1916 Dr.Leys ordered the Sisters to go to Mwaya in Tanganyika, because of the fighting there. Sr.Jacques wrote "quite a number killed and wounded. After two months at Karonga, we disembarked at the extreme end of the Lake in conquered territory. The English had established the military hospital there."

September 16th 1916 Mwaya "As a bird on the branch, I have no fixed abode. A small house of reeds was started for us. In the meantime we were given lodging and dined with the Nurses. These ladies were charming and told us to say our prayers together as it would not disturb them. In less than a week our African reed monastery was ready, four small rooms and a chapel."

The Nyasaland Field Force employed 169,000 carriers to take supplies to the front line. Seven major hospitals were set up, each in charge of a doctor, with over a hundred medical dressers. Sister Jaques wrote "these poor Africans have a hard life, carrying provisions of food and ammunition for 25 miles in the blazing sun is exhausting. No wonder that at the end of 7 or 8 months they come to the end of their strength. We have seen several die. Please ask our Sisters to pray for these dear souls. They find it very strange that we wash them, tend their wounds, and, if need arises, feed them like children."

December 8th 1916 "We have been ordered to leave Mwaya and go to Old Langenburg where hundreds of sick await attention. On November 12th we boarded the *Gwendolen* with all the equipment of our mobile hospital, to cross the Lake and take up residence in the hilly country.

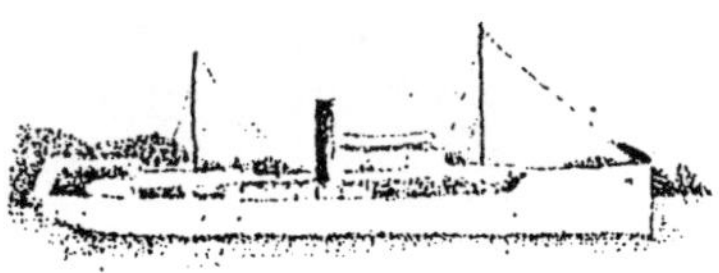

Gwendolen

We were quite surprised to find a hut ready to receive us, and a large room able to shelter 120 patients under the command of Major Dr.Hugh Stannus. Our house resembles a Trappist monastery with an austere grille of bamboo, but we have a wonderful view of the Lake. The country is arid and hot like Utale. We are the only daughters of Eve in the area. About 25 European men are employed for transport, and a few thousand African carriers of foodstuffs and ammunition to the soldiers. Camp life is good for us and we (Sr.Jaques and Sr.Reine) are both well; slight doses of fever and other small unavoidable incidents with our life on the move do not darken our spiritual horizon. We are happy with whatever Divine Providence sends us daily. Bless your two vagabond Sisters in the African Bush."

January 1917 "The hospital is always crowded. A big thankyou for the parcel sent; I wait expectantly for the clothes for I am not alone in mine (even in my suspenders these unwelcome hosts lodge). This does not mean that the

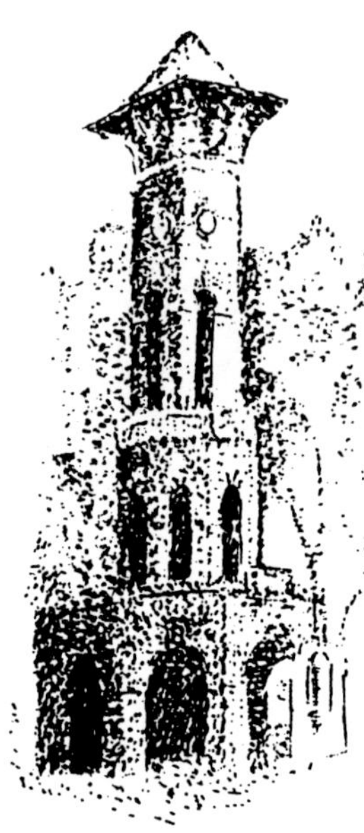

King's African Rifles.
War Memorial Zomba.
W.W.1
African dead
from wounds 735
from disease 481
British dead 127

mangoes, coming with them, will not also be gratefully received. Thankyou for everything."

February 18th 1917 "If this campaign lasts much longer, I am afraid of becoming a pagan! Our hospital is so crowded, dysentery is epidemic, and many others have fever. To crown it all Plague has broken out. The Germans, with 1,200 Askaris and 6 white men, with 2 cannons and 15 machine guns came to Old Langenburg. Father put up Red Cross flags over the hospital. Twice yesterday the telegraph wire was cut and the Captain has no news."

February 25th 1917 "The wounded continue to arrive, the battle is raging a few miles from here, the machine guns and cannons thunder, and shots whistle without stop. Old Langenburg is in a state of siege, and facing the hospital is a small boat, on which the cannon is pointed at the mouth of the Lumbira River. The sentinels posted on the mountains surrounding the small town keep a strong watch. Over the hospital and our humble dwelling the Red Cross flag is flying. Vain precautions, for our trust is in Our Lady. Amid the storm there are serene and happy days for us and our poor patients."

August 12th 1917 "General Northey appreciates and thanks us for the good care we take of the carriers and soldiers. He speaks French well so it is easy for us to welcome him."

"We have had to leave Old Langenburg to follow the army, so here we are at Ilala, still on the shores of Lake Nyasa. The camp is situated on a sea of sand, which is extremely hot. On arriving I had fever for a few days but my companion (Sr.Reine) is wonderfully cheerful and well. Two of us (Sr.Reine and I) are called to the camp at Penamiho. Fighting is fierce and the wounded are numerous. Penamiho is a Catholic Mission where there were two Benedictine Priests and seven Religious Sisters. Fr.Martin has again followed the troops, to give first aid to the wounded, and then direct them to the hospital at the rear." "Work is not lacking, all human misery meets us here in our mobile hospital, I regret not being able to describe each ward; there is one for each sickness from mental illness to elephantiasis. Some facts could be related by a more expert hand."

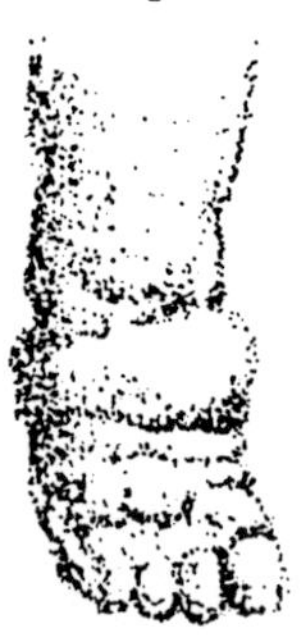

Elephantiasis

January 6th 1918 Mother Provincial writes from Nguludi "I wish that Sister du Sauveur, after two years of camp life, could come here, so that we could renew their supply of linen and any other needs. There is a rumour that Sr.Jacques and her companion Sr. Reine, who, it is said, get through piles of work, have come 50 miles nearer. The scene of

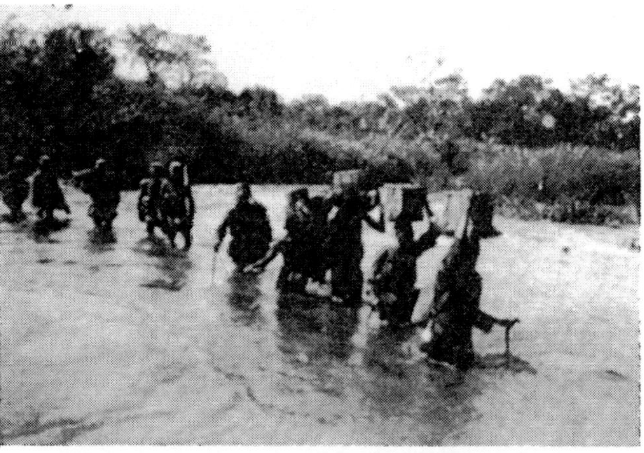

Tenga-tenga (carriers) and troops. 500 mile march 1918.

military action has changed, the Germans have escaped into Portuguese Mozambique."

August 1918 at Fort Johnston Military Hospital "Here we are again in Nyasaland, two days distance from Blantyre, Nzama, and Utale. From these Missions we have received fruit and vegetables. How sweet and appreciated is this sisterly kindness which unites the houses of our Shire Mission. One day a basket of oranges, the next a sack of beans and green vegetables."

Major Dr.Chisholm from Mwenzo station of the Livingstonia Mission was in command of Fort Johnston hospital, "his wife, who is very amiable, is a nurse. She accompanies her husband to the hospital and often visits us."

"Sr.Reine and I are at the Bar which is at the end of the Lake where the boats dock. Our wards are 30 yards from our hut, with 140 African patients suffering from typhoid, malaria or dysentery; a few cases of smallpox, and many wounds to tend. We care for the souls as well as the bodies of our poor patients. In the evening we rest from the day's fatigue, kneeling near the Blessed Sacrament."

"The Anglican nurses from Malindi Mission invited us to visit and prepared a real English 5 o'clock tea for us. Cakes and dainties, nothing was lacking. But this luxury made me love our frugal life with only biscuits or fruits to offer these gentlemen who call in when passing to greet the missionaries."

September 4th 1918 The Order recorded "Sr.Jacques was in bed with a temperature of 103° F. She was red or crimson

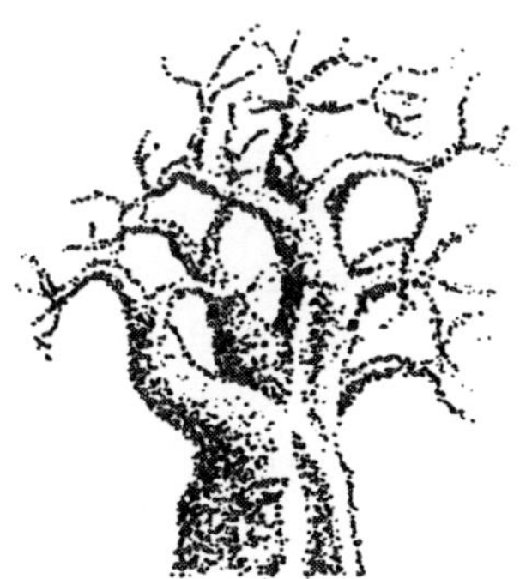

Lakeside Baobab

purple, her face swollen, she could not quench her thirst, not ease her interior burning. Dr.Chisholm came to see her morning and evening. Smallpox was suspected because our dear Sister had cared for patients with this dangerous sickness. She had a few spots on her body, but these marks did not get larger nor red. Sr.Reine and I, taking every possible precaution, cared for her night and day, because the poor patient could not sleep."

Saturday September 7th 1918 "The thermometer read 105° F, after a restless night, her thirst increased, the poor patient's face was swollen, her eyes bloodshot, and her tonsils so enlarged that she could hardly swallow. She said 'I cannot speak properly,".

Sunday September 8th 1918 "The fever dropped, replaced by freezing interior cold; she asked to be covered and longed for a hot drink, but nothing made us think of the approaching end. We attended Mass, on the other side of the reed partition. The patient called and complained of being cold...though conscious she could not make herself understood. Father started the anointing, when our good Sister gave up her soul to God.

Dr.Chisholm came immediately, all surprised and sorrowful. The body blackened quickly, so he ordered an immediate funeral." All the people of Fort Johnston, the Commander of the Army, the Officers, and the troops, accompanied this dear departed Sister. "The soldiers presented arms, and now a fervent Daughter of Wisdom is the first Catholic to be buried in Fort Johnston military cemetery." (Opposite modern Mangochi Hospital).

> *Mother Sister Salvator*
> *Nyasaland Nursing Service*
> *8th September 1918.*

CATHOLIC HOSPITALS
The Montfort Fathers

Nguludi Hospital originated in a small dispensary in 1903. Brother Tarcisco and Brother Gerard supervised the hospital building after 1950. The Nursing School has flourished with good results in qualifying examinations.*

Another venture has been the **School for the Deaf** started by Brother Hortensius with financial support from the Commonwealth Foundation. It trains teachers of the Deaf from several African countries and has an international reputation. There is also a **Blind School**.

Phalombe Hospital was founded by the Medical Mission Sisters in 1960, opening in three rooms. The first was the outpatient dispensary, the second had a few beds for in-patients, and the third was occupied by the Sisters. Construction of a proper hospital began a year later, and the Hospital soon trained nurses.

*Illus.p.139

Mlambe Hospital was started by three Dutch Sisters in Lunzu town in 1963. The Chapel is an architectural gem, and open to visitors.

At **Trinity** Hospital and School of Nursing at Muona, on the east bank of the Shire River, the Sisters of Divine Providence have pioneered outreach services to remote areas, where malnutrition is a problem.

At **Nchalo**, Sisters started a mobile unit in 1967, dispensing care to 70 villages in the lands around the Elephant Marsh. Mud huts and bush schools served as their dispensaries. "The biggest problem was our habit, the white was very impractical in the dusty roads and dirt huts we worked in. Laundry was a real problem...in many villages we met with indifference and suspicion, yet we continue to visit." Their work grew, and soon a hospital was needed. This now serves the large Sucoma sugar estate.

Utale Mission offered care to leprosy patients for many years after a ward was opened in the 1930s.

In 1962, the Federal Government authorized 153 Montfort hospital beds, and 660 White Father beds, for government grants. The intention of Catholic hospitals has been to provide services in more isolated areas. Outreach pioneering health work has been a special feature of the Catholic endeavour. They are now directed by the local Malawian Catholic Church with considerable outside financial help.

White Fathers

Likuni Mission opened a dispensary in 1941 and patients had to pay a fee - "What is given free is not appreciated" wrote the Bishop. Sister Trinitas-Koop from Holland served for 50 years as a White Sister at Likuni hospital, starting with five mud huts in 1940. She devised the famous phala (thin porridge) for malnourished children that is now used all over Africa. It consists of: groundnuts 25%, beans 25%, and maize 50%.

Mua Mission opened a leprosy ward in 1927. In the 1930s maternal and child health units were started at Mtakataka and Mua. After World War II this work expanded and a hospital was built. There are also hospitals at Namitete, Madisi, Namwera, and Kasina.

In 1962, **St. John's** Hospital at Mzuzu was started by the Medical Mission Sisters of Mary. It now has 200 beds, and a School of Nursing with 60 nurse/ midwives. Today it serves the rapidly growing city of Mzuzu. Mobile clinic services in the Northern Region of Malaŵi are also provided.

24 THE FEDERATION OF RHODESIA AND NYASALAND 1953-64

In 1953, the Nyasaland health budget was greatly increased with revenue from the then rich economies of Northern and Southern Rhodesia, now Zambia and Zimbabwe. A local doctor commented "in colonial days there was a lot of sympathy for the health services, but little money. During the Federation, medical supplies and staff became generously available." A mission nurse was more explicit: "the amalgamation of the three Territories brought one great blessing: drugs, hitherto rationed and meagre, now flowed in a steady stream. No longer was it necessary to weigh up the pros and cons of a severe illness, wondering whether this was the one to receive the precious penicillin, or whether to give it to a more deserving case. We could now save the lives of many who had been doomed to die."

With more money, more staff could be employed, and facilities improved. An extensive hospital building programme was effected during the Federation in all regions of Nyasaland. For instance, in 1959, "substantial additions were made to the wards at Kasungu District hospital, a 50 bed hospital is being built at Chinteche, and an 86 bed hospital has been built at Nkhata Bay. Liwonde Rural Hospital has been virtually reconstructed, and Balaka and Kaluluma Hospitals put into service. Another rural hospital at Mwanza is ready."

Special maternity wards were added to all the bigger hospitals, X-Ray plants installed, proper houses for staff were built, very many rural health centres were constructed. Primary health care was pioneered with funds for antenatal clinics, underfives clinics, and immunization policies.

However, a good service created its own demand, and in 1957 it was reported "the bed provision in government hospitals is 1,797 and the daily average number of patients is 1,833, an overcrowding index of 102." The number of beds per thousand people in Nyasaland was 5·6 in 1958.

GOVERNMENT HOSPITALS					
	1955	1962		1955	1962
Hospital	Beds	Beds	Hospital	Beds	Beds
Blantyre	63	397	Karonga	44	44
Chikwawa	40	68	Kasungu	48	77
Chiradzulu	45	78	Nkhota Kota	123	140
Chinteche	54	54	Lilongwe	153	203
Thyolo	61	132	Mulanje	71	100
Dedza	50	51	Mzimba	60	132
Dowa	41	99	Ntcheu	49	53
Mangochi	73	107	Chiromo	50	103
Mchinji	40	76	Zomba	194	282

The major building was The Queen Elizabeth Hospital in Blantyre, which was opened by Queen Elizabeth the Queen Mother in 1958. Modern medical facilities were provided, and patients of all races from all districts of Nyasaland could now be referred for investigation and treatment by specialists. The building design is attractive for patients and staff. The wards are linked by long corridors. The local newspaper reported "Matron will tour the Queen Elizabeth Hospital on a bicycle" and "the £750,000 hospital can take 412 beds without overcrowding."

A fuller range of doctors was appointed during the Federation, many coming from Southern Rhodesia. There were Specialists in Surgery, Medicine, Ophthalmology, Pathology, Radiology, TB, Obstetrics, and Psychiatry.

The future leader of Malaŵi returned in 1958.

THE LIFE PRESIDENT OF THE REPUBLIC OF MALAŴI

Ngwazi Dr. H. Kamuzu Banda

He first went to school under a Kachere tree near his birthplace at Mtunthama near Kasungu. The school was run by Church of Scotland Presbyterian Missionaries. Because there were no opportunities for further education in his own country, he felt compelled even at the young age of 13 years, to walk more than 1,600 kilometres to the Republic of South Africa for further training.

He eventually enrolled at Meharry Medical College in Nashville, Tennessee, U.S.A., where he qualified as a doctor in 1937. Kamuzu Banda then travelled to Britain and continued his studies in medicine at Edinburgh University. During the war years of 1939-45 he practised Medicine in Liverpool and North Shields. In 1945 he moved to London. In 1953 he left England for Ghana where he established a medical practice in Kumasi.

Dr. H. Kamuzu Banda returned to Nyasaland on 6th July 1958 and led the struggle for independence. He became Nyasaland's first Prime Minister in 1963. In 1966 he became the first President of the Republic of Malaŵi.

Training of medical assistants, nurses, and midwives, took place at Blantyre, Zomba, and Lilongwe. A blood transfusion service was started in Blantyre in 1961, with the Red Cross collecting blood. Considerable expansion of the Mission Hospitals took place - at Namitete a new Catholic hospital of 88 beds, and a new 60 bed hospital at Livingstonia, were opened. In 1961 it was reported "Missions are finding that the resources in men and money they used to be able to call on from Europe are now diminishing." Resources though were readily supplied from local finances within the federated territories.

1962 Medical Mission beds authorized for government grants	
Church of Scotland	228
Dutch Reformed Church	302
Catholic Church	813
Baptists	17
Adventists	96
Universities Mission	143

However, the Federation was not a happy time in the Nation's history. The gap in understanding between European administrators and African villagers became obvious in the well meaning attempts to introduce immunization programmes and to control disease. Poor and ignorant people fled from the smallpox vaccinators when they reached a village, polio vaccines lay stored in refrigerators as parents declined it for their children, the WHO residual spraying programme for malarial mosquitoes in Zomba, Blantyre, and Lake Chilwa area had to be abandoned because of lack of co-operation from the local people.

In 1960, the WHO tuberculosis assessment team had to withdraw before even a little information could be gathered. It had not been understood that it is the patient's privilege to decide what medical help he or she wants, and people living in ignorance and poverty could not understand the nature of the disease.

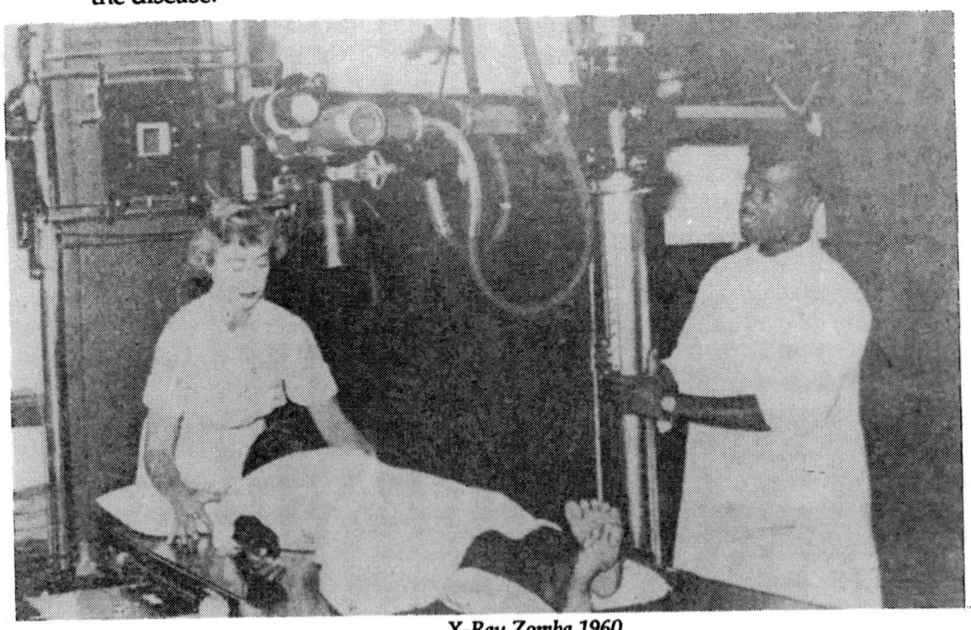

X-Ray Zomba 1960

The last years of the Federation were a sad time for the morale of the health services. The old Nysasland medical staff were required to transfer to the Federal Service by 1959, or resign. Only 12 of the 40 expatriate doctors did so, and only 3 of the 34 senior staff. There was a great reluctance on the part of local Malaŵian staff to transfer. The epilogue of the Federal Health Service can be quoted from the final Annual Report:

1958 The Federation of Rhodesia and Nyasaland	Southern Rhodesia	Northern Rhodesia	Nyasaland
Population total	2,770,000	2,300,000	2,710,000
European	207,000	72,000	8,300
Size (square miles)	150,000	290,000	46,000
Health expenditure			
1953	£2,202,000	£1,091,000	£273,000
1958	£3,655,000	£2,170,000	£715,000
Medical officers			
1953	95	60	38
1958	116	78	46
Trained nurses			
1953	475	151	34
1958	718	303	57
African admissions to Government hospitals			
1953	324,000	118,000	34,000
1958	475,000	151,000	64,000
African outpatients			
1953	1,892,000	2,197,000	1,209,000
1958	3,090,000	5,611,000	4,217,000

"The Federal Ministry withered at the end of 1962, and 1963, had to be spent in preparing for dissolution. It can justly be claimed that the Federal Government, in its nearly 10 years of life, gave a great impetus and drive to the development of health and medical services of the Federation which must contribute greatly to the future development of the territorial services."

However, in the last days, the number of government doctors dropped to 14, and medical stores were taken back to Rhodesia. As the table shows, Nyasaland, although undoubtedly benefitting in health matters, always remained a poor relation in the Federation.

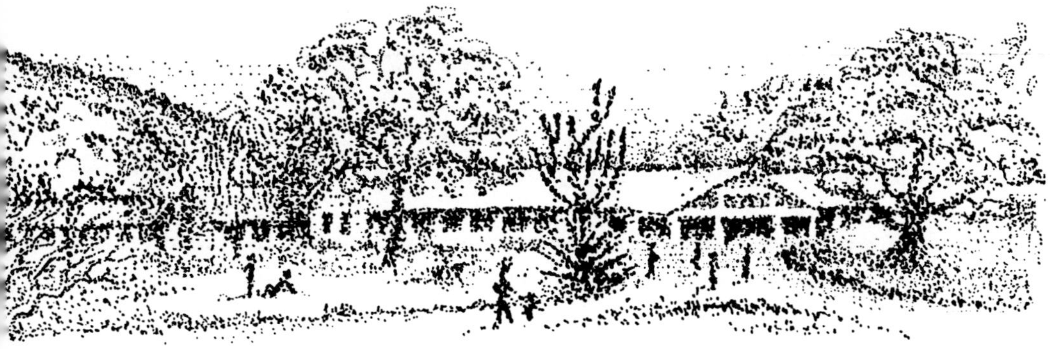

Queen Elizabeth Hospital, Blantyre.

25 INDEPENDENT MALAŴI

The outlook for the services in the country, as the Federation of Rhodesia and Nyasaland was breaking up, did not look healthy. In the year before Independence on 6th July 1964, there was a handing over period. At one time there were only 14 doctors (one Malaŵian) in the government service, 13 posts were vacant, and medical stores were being taken to Rhodesia. However, in response to a request from the Government, the Israelis sent 8 doctors, and extra staff came from Britain, Holland, and 11 other countries within a few years. Two Malaŵian newly qualified doctors returned from India in the year of Independence, one, Dr.D. Chilemba was later to become Chief Medical Officer.

The Medical Association of Malaŵi was formed in 1964 and had a membership of 27 (including mission and private doctors). The hope that the 32 Malaŵian medical students training abroad (mainly in Britain, but also in Uganda, India, and South Africa) would return by 1969 was unfortunately not realized, although the number of Malaŵian doctors rose from 3 in 1964 to 12 in 1972. There has been a poor return from other doctor training schemes, and today, about 25 of the 175 doctors in the country are Malaŵian. There are more than twice that number outside the country. The majority of the expatriate doctors are from Holland, Britain, and other European countries, with some from U.S.A. and Japan. They are usually partially funded by various Aid schemes. The country has a total of 35 Specialists, and there is a sizeable group of Malaŵian Asians among the 23 General Practitioners. There are 17 Dentists in the country compared with 3 at Independence.

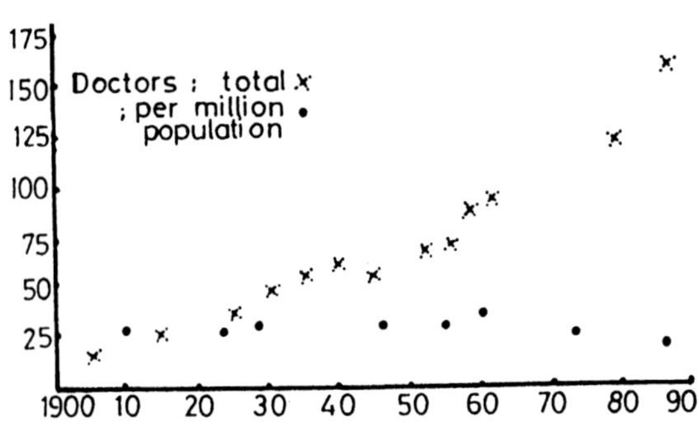

The Private Hospital Association of Malaŵi PHAM was formed in 1965 and today consists of 15 different denominations running 21 hospitals, 38 primary health care centres, 76 health sub-centres, and 13 training schools. Since 1978, the Government has subsidized the salaries of the Malaŵian staff working in PHAM units. The Mission hospitals make a small charge for services. The Government services are free, although there is provision for private paying facilities at some hospitals.

The Malaŵi Council for the Handicapped MACOHA was set up with the help of the International Labour Organization. Vocational training is given at Magomero, in the same area as the UMCA Mission of 1861. There is an impressive weaving factory for the handicapped at Limbe, and tie-dye workshop in Lilongwe.

In 1980 the highly regarded Medical Quarterly was started by Dr M.E.Molyneux.

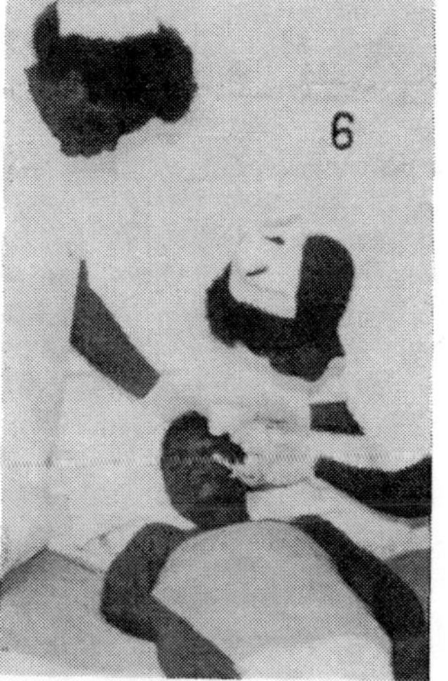

In the early 1960s, 112 Malaŵian student nurses were sent overseas for training, and the National School of Nursing was opened with 25 students in 1965. The last government expatriate nursing sisters and matrons left in 1976. Today 60 State Registered Nurse Midwives and 265 State Enrolled Nurse Midwives are training annually in the country.

The Clinical Officers, Medical Assistants, Radiography, Pharmacy, and Laboratory, Assistants are trained in Lilongwe and Blantyre.

In the first 10 years of Independence the staff of the Ministry increased by 50% and recurrent expenditure doubled (80% on curative, 8% on preventive, medicine). The number of staff has continued to increase, 1,750 in 1974 to 5,800 in 1987. However this number should almost double by 1996 if the service is to be adequately staffed, taking into account the population increases. It is unlikely there are adequate resources and training facilities to achieve this. The Health share of the national budget for the last 20 years has been around 7 - 8%. This amounts to K6·5 per head per year.(£1·30, US $2·30))

Since Independence, 12 new or improved and enlarged hospitals have been built. Most have been commissioned within the last decade, and funded by the European Economic Community, or by British, German, and Danish, Aid, or with loans from International Agencies.

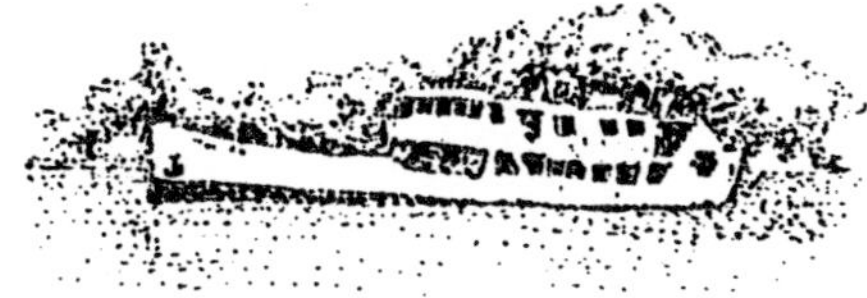

The Chauncy Maples after conversion to diesel by Malawi Railways in 1965. She was built in Glasgow in 1899, reassembled on the Lake and used for many years by the U.M.C.A. Still sailing today.

STAFF 1980	
Government Doctors	54
PHAM Doctors	37
Private Doctors	30
Total number of Doctors	121
Senior Clinical Officers	46
Clinical Officers	61
Medical Assistants	547
S.R.N.M.	402
S.E.N.M.	1,293

BEDS 1986		
Government Hospitals	24	4,120
PHAM Hospitals	20	2,722
Primary Health Care Centres	38	1,459
Dispensary/Maternity Units	164	962
Maternity Units	96	351
Dispensaries	310	303
Health Posts	67	8

The increase in the population, coupled with the confidence in the health services, has led to a big demand, so hospitals and outpatient clinics are crowded. In spite of this, the Malaŵian patient is more fortunate than those in many African hospitals. The staff are cheerful and hard working, and essential drugs and materials usually are available. It is appropriate that in the 1991 Centenary Year of the definition of the country's borders, the first group of 14 medical students have returned from Britain for their final year in the new Medical College of Malaŵi.

1986 Kamuzu Central Hospital, Lilongwe

Right: Top ten causes of adult medical admissions. Total 2,788.

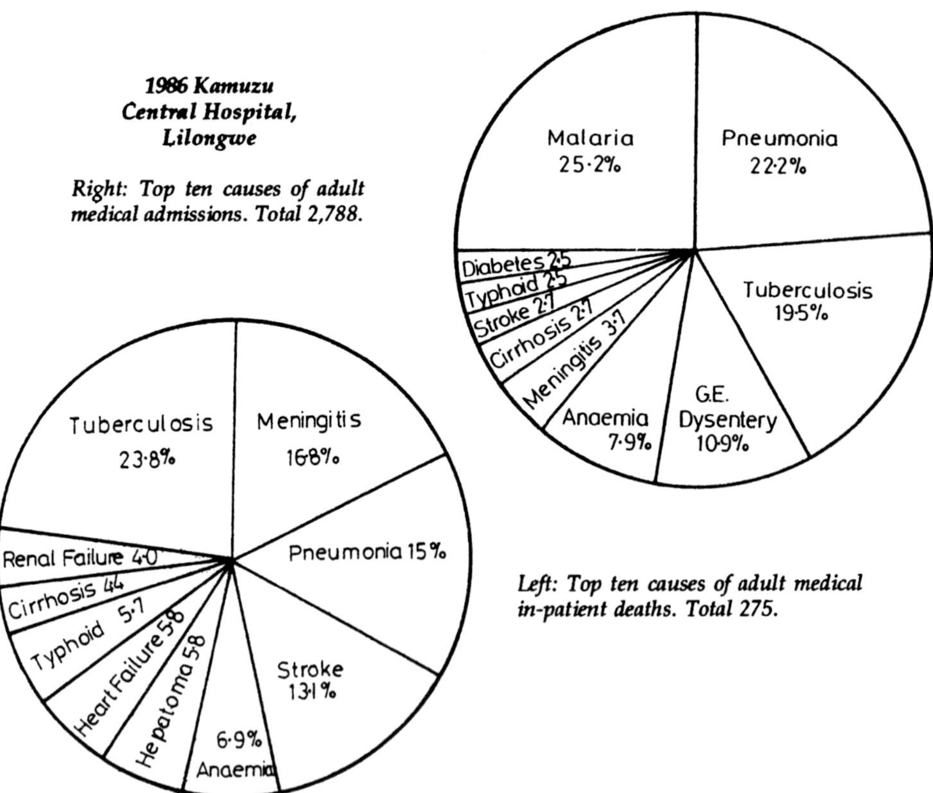

Left: Top ten causes of adult medical in-patient deaths. Total 275.

<table>
<tr><td colspan="4" align="center">STAFF 1990</td></tr>
<tr><td>Doctors</td><td>175</td><td>Radiography Assistants</td><td>34</td></tr>
<tr><td>(35 Specialists)</td><td></td><td>Laboratory Technicians</td><td>55</td></tr>
<tr><td>Clinical Officers</td><td>221</td><td>Laboratory Assistants</td><td>52</td></tr>
<tr><td>Medical Assistants</td><td>501</td><td>State Registered Nurses</td><td>75</td></tr>
<tr><td>Dentists</td><td>17</td><td>SRN + Midwifery</td><td>485</td></tr>
<tr><td>Dental Technicians</td><td>8</td><td>State Enrolled Nurses</td><td>70</td></tr>
<tr><td>Physiotherapists</td><td>17</td><td>SEN + Midwifery</td><td>1,780</td></tr>
<tr><td>Radiographers</td><td>6</td><td>Midwives</td><td>199</td></tr>
</table>

Since 1986, increasing numbers of refugees from the Mozambique war have crossed into Malaŵi, especially in the South and around Dedza. There are an estimated 850,000, or 10% of the population, and the numbers are increasing by several hundred each week. In the Nsanje area they outnumber the local inhabitants by 20%. Dr. Grace Malenga (Paediatrician) one of the first Malawian woman doctors, is now the U.N.H.C.R. Health Co-ordinator. Malaŵi's policy of an open door welcome has been supported by International Aid but is stressing the land, water, and health resources in many areas.

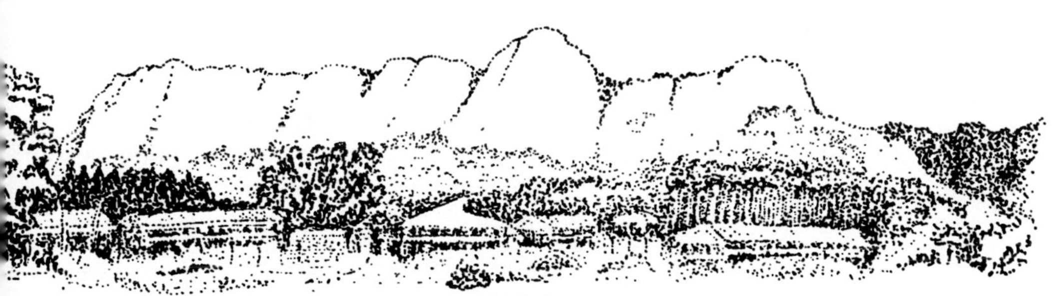

New Mulanje Hospital built by E.E.C.(1992)

Viruses are minute agents that can only grow and multiply within a living cell. Smallpox, hepatitis, influenza, measles, are viral illnesses. The body can develop immunity after exposure to the disease or the killed or modified virus in a vaccine. There is no general antibiotic against them as yet.

Aids is a devastating new plague sweeping the world with no vaccine or cure. It directly attacks the body's immune system. Polio is an ancient disease with an effective vaccine and it is possible it could be eliminated from the world as smallpox has been.

POLIO

The wasted contracted limbs of Infantile Paralysis, the old term for Poliomyelitis, were easily recognized and noted by pioneer doctors. The acute phase of the disease is not easily diagnosed except in epidemics. In 1925, 495 cases were reported with no deaths (probably only a fraction of all cases were diagnosed and reported).

In 1954, 26 African and 5 European cases were reported and the differences between the groups commented upon. The Europeans were young adults and severely affected by paralysis, whereas in the Africans it was a relatively mild disease in children under five years. This is because the virus, which attacks the spinal cord, is spread via the intestinal route (faecal/oral transmission). Where there is poor hygiene, babies come early into contact with the virus when they are still protected by maternal antibodies, and probably develop a degree of immunity.

Even today there is no antibiotic that can kill the virus and prevention by vaccination is necessary. The Salk injection vaccine was available in Nyasaland in 1957, but often parents were unwilling to bring their children. However, in that year there was a severe polio outbreak in Southern Africa with 81 cases reported in Nyasaland. In 1959, only 1,669 doses were issued, but two years later there was a marked increase in the

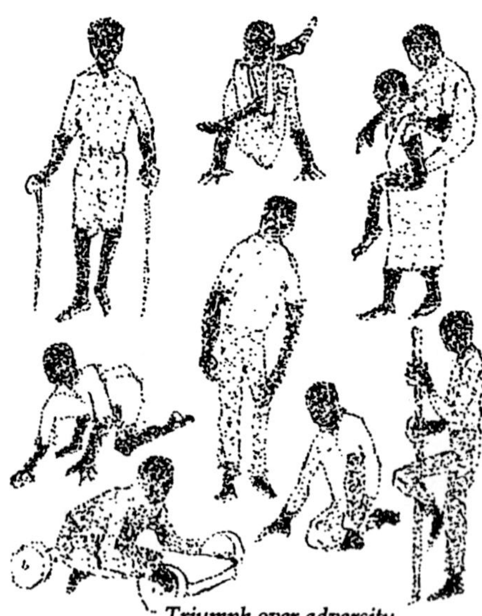

Triumph over adversity.
Polio Vioctims before M.A.P.

number of cases and a vaccination campaign was started. The oral Sabin vaccine then became available.

In 1979 the Save the Children Fund (S.C.F.) carried out a survey in Malawi. It was estimated that 6·5 per 1,000 surviving children under 10 years had residual paralysis from Polio, usually of the legs. This was 17,500 out of the 2·5 million children in this age group. 14% of these would be severely affected and unable to walk, another 14% would need sticks and callipers to walk around.

The S.C.F. instituted the Stop Polio campaign on a national scale with the co-operation of the Health services and the local Chiefs and officials. The main problem was keeping the live oral vaccine cool enough, so preserving its potency up to the time it was delivered in remote villages. The campaign was very successful with most children receiving the three doses required. Polio vaccine is part of the regular extended immunization programme for children (E.P.I.), and fresh cases are rarely seen in Malawi today. However there are large numbers of physically disabled remaining from old polio and other causes, estimated at 50,000 in 1978. Until recently the hard pressed health services could do little for them, until Malawi Against Polio was formed.

M.A.P. Malawi Against Polio.

Wasted contracted limbs can be straightened by operation and strengthened with external metal callipers and crutches. The mobility of severely affected patients can be improved by giving them a wheelchair. M.A.P. was formed to do this in 1979 by the chief surgeon, Dr.J.A. Borgstein, and the Archbishop of Central Africa, Donald Arden. Outside help came from Professor Ronald Huckstep, an orthopaedic surgeon who had previously set up a low cost, appropriate technology, polio help programme in Uganda.

By 1980, Rotary International had given U.S. $ 250,000 and staff had been recruited. Over the past decade, with the co-operation of the Ministry of Health, more and more clinics have been opened in the remote rural areas. Now

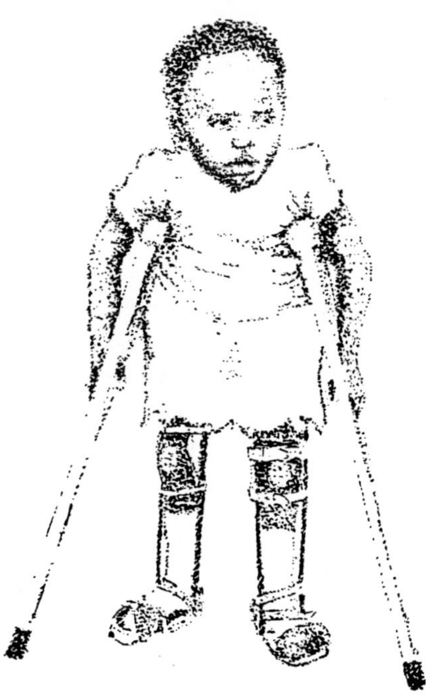

there are more than 80 clinics and they receive monthly visits by the team (usually a physiotherapist and a workman to repair appliances, sometimes a doctor). In 1988/89, 21,167 patients were seen, 572 operations carried out, many by visiting volunteer orthopaedic surgeons, and 18,000 appliances issued, made in the four M.A.P. workshops.

M.A.P. is a charity and relies on funding from Oxfam, the Commissioner of the European Communities, Christoffel Blinden Mission, and other external agencies, as well as enthusiastic local fundraising. Memisa Medicus Mundi, U.S. Peace Corps, and British Volunteer Services Overseas provide some professional staff.

Today, in spite of its name, under a third of patients have polio, the rest suffer from talipes (club foot, common in Africa), cerebral palsy (a result of birth trauma or cerebral malaria), and various disabling conditions (bone injury and infections, and burns).

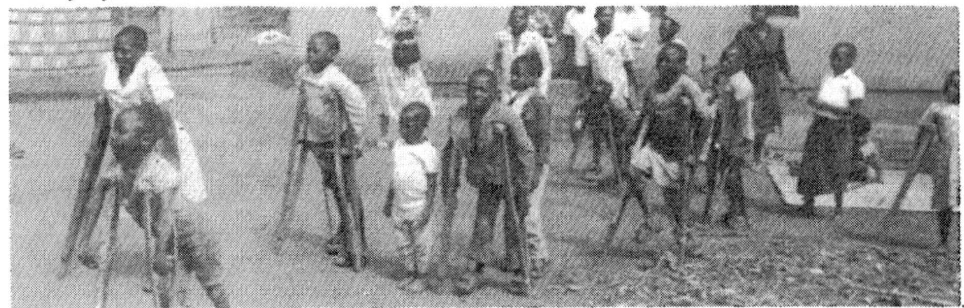

Patients at the Rumphi clinic.

AIDS Acquired Immune Deficiency Syndrome

In Malaŵi in the mid 1980s, a change in the character of some cases of Kaposi's Sarcoma was noticed. This was usually a slow growing nodular skin tumour of the legs, but it seemed to be presenting in a more aggressive way, and in unusual sites. At the same time, in the medical wards, an increasing number of young, urban, patients were admitted with weight loss, unusual infections, and enlarged lymph nodes.

In 1985 Aids testing became possible, and it was shown that these patients had Aids Related Complexes (ARC), and were infected by the Human Immunodeficiency Virus (HIV). Small surveys showed a 2% HIV positive rate in otherwise fit pregnant mothers in the ante-natal clinics, and in blood donors. This figure rose to 8% in 1987, 19% in 1989, and to 23% in an urban ante-natal centre in 1990.

Some rural areas surveyed have a much lower rate. The wards of hospitals have increasing numbers of Aids patients, putting strains on the health services and nursing staff. Over a quarter of hospital beds are occupied by ARC patients. Aids is a fatal condition. In some hospitals in Africa and in Malawi it is becoming the main cause of death.

Aids was first recorded in the U.S.A. in 1981 among homosexuals and drug abusers. The virus was identified in 1983, and tests for the antibody to the virus have improved over the years. The largest accumulation of cases is in East and Central Africa. There are equal numbers of males and females affected. In Malawi, as in the

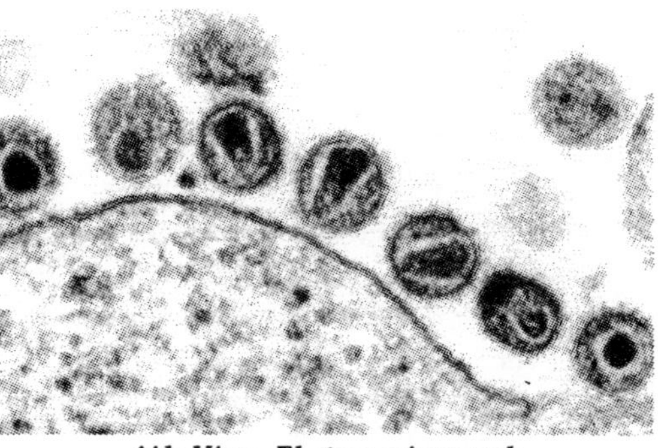
Aids Virus. Electron micrograph

surrounding countries, women are affected at a younger age. Between the ages of 15 and 19 years, 85% of the Aids patients are women. Men predominate over 30 years. The disease is spread heterosexually, probably helped by the high incidence of genital sores.

Blood donations are screened in Malawi, and needles and instruments are sterilized. Patients and relatives are generally counselled. There is an Aids Control programme supported by WHO, and run by Dr. N.G.Liomba, the first Malawian pathologist. As in several badly affected countries, this programme has only a limited impact. There is a section of the population aged 5-15 years that is free of Aids, and this is the most worthwhile group to concentrate on, with teaching and information.

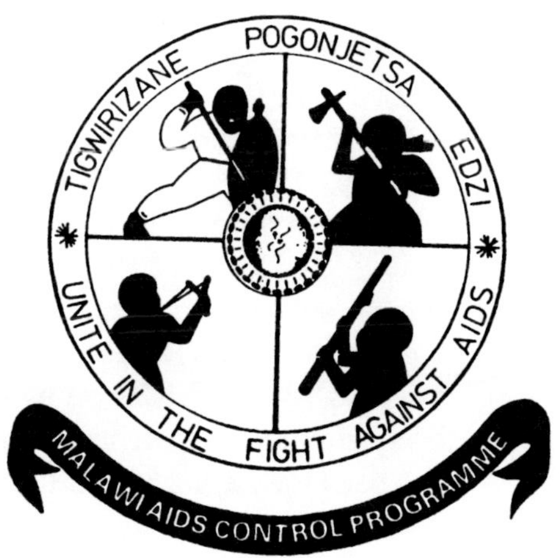

The fate of babies born to HIV mothers is being studied in Blantyre. Not all apparently get Aids, but it is an increasingly common cause of infant death. Aids will be the most serious test of the health services yet, and may have long reaching effects on the social structure of the nation. It is however easy to avoid catching Aids. A person with only one Aids-free sexual partner will not catch this disease.

27 MOTHER AND CHILD

MATERNITY SERVICES

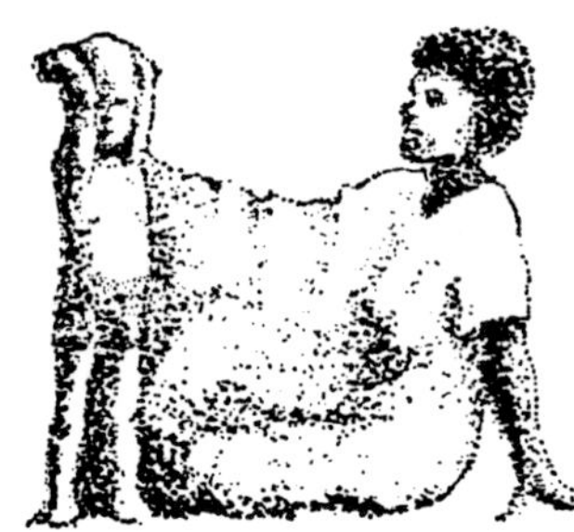

Life sized terra-cotta statue at Queen Elizabeth Hospital Blantyre.

In 1890, Dr.George Steele*, newly arrived from Glasgow, wrote at Njuyu in Chief M'mbelwa's Ngoni area: "About four weeks ago I was called to one of the Chief's villages to a complicated labour case. All went well. The gratitude of the people was very sincere. The women came round me on their knees, slowly clapping their hands, and saying in a tone of great relief 'Baba be, Baba be'(our Father), a term of great respect." This is one of the first recorded maternity cases in this country.

It was an uncommon medical event. For another half century childbirth was managed almost entirely by traditional birth attendants in the villages. Occasionally help was sought. In 1896, Dr.Prentice at Bandawe noted: "Towards the end of the year we had quite a number of complicated obstetric cases, and were often able to render life-saving aid." At Karonga in 1910, Dr. Innes said "obstetric work also has its place resulting in the saving of lives." This probably reflects the excellent clinical qualities of these doctors. Patients were attracted by a good service. Obstetric cases were absent from many other hospitals, including those staffed by women.

At Mvera in 1910, Dr.William Murray had many maternity patients, and he actually trained the first local midwife, Sara Nabanda. In 1928, another Murray, Dr.Pauline Murray, started the first midwifery school at Mlanda Mission, high up in the mountains at Lisulu. "More abnormal midwifery is encountered there than at our larger hospitals; and as the population, largely Ngoni, seems to be more hospital minded than some other areas, there is enough teaching material. Ngoni matrons are also conservative in their attitude towards young girls as midwives. Until now only married women have been admitted as students. As the standard of girls' education in the country has been low, it has been difficult to find women of the necessary status as useful village midwives, and at the same time who are more than merely literate." By 1934, an average of 40 mothers were delivering in Mlanda hospital each year, and six midwives who had completed the training course, were working in surrounding villages.

The Scottish Missions started midwifery courses at Bandawe hospital

* *Illus. inside front cover*

(7 confinements in 1933), and at Blantyre under Dr.Janet Welch in 1932. Six young widows were training as midwives. Traditionally widows attended childbirth. The reported mortality rates were then high. In 134 deliveries at Blantyre in 1933, there were 11 maternal deaths and 41 babies were born dead. By 1935, 25% of the mothers in abnormal labour died, and 9% of the children were born dead.

In 1928, the Jeanes Institute at Domasi near Zomba was set up with a female staff to pioneer rural maternity services. Chief Malemia and his wife attended the classes and tried to persuade local women to seek obstetric help. However the number of confinements at the Jeanes remained very low (only 2 per month after 8 years). In 1936 the Jeanes Report noted "the root of the trouble is the deeply held fears and tribal taboos of the uneducated village women. Only after much propaganda and demonstration of results can a real impression be made." The Jeanes described two maternal deaths. One woman had been in labour for 5 days prior to admission and died before delivery, the second death occurred three days after craniotomy for contracted pelvis.

It was the advent of Obstetric Surgery that transformed the maternity scene here. In 1936 two Scottish surgeons arrived. Mr.C.H. Howat F.R.C.S.(Edin) was posted to Fort Johnston, and Mr.H.D. Cronyn F.R.C.S.(Edin) went to Zomba. The first recorded Caesarian operation in this country was soon performed by Mr.Cronyn under spinal anaesthesia: "among the abnormal midwifery cases were three patients who required Caesarian section, curiously the three cases occurred in the same month." (1936)

The news soon spread that the lives of mothers and babies could now be saved by surgeons, and hundreds of maternity patients came to these hospitals. By 1943, 2,000 women were admitted to Government hospitals for delivery, and a year later the numbers doubled. In 1946 a Government Midwives' Board was set up, with a national two year course and standard examinations.

Hospital Confinements	
1948	6,745
1949	7,742
1950	6,892
1951	9,804

During the Federation, maternity wards were added to the bigger hospitals with much improved surgical facilities. The first Specialist Obstetrician was appointed in 1961. There has been a large demand for maternity services in Independent Malawi.The maternal mortality rate is nevertheless one of the highest in Africa, estimated at 17 per 1,000 deliveries in 1984. The risks to the woman's health and life increase with the number of pregnancies. The very high birth rate, and the consequent rapid increase in population has overstressed the obstetric services.

Expansion of crowded wards was soon needed. In 1980 the Life President of Malawi, donated the fine modern Maternity Unit at the Queen Elizabeth Hospital, Blantyre. Excellent modern surgical facilities are provided. In 1989, there were 1,128 Caesarian operations performed in this Maternity Unit. In 1982, modern family planning was integrated into the Maternal and Child Health Services.

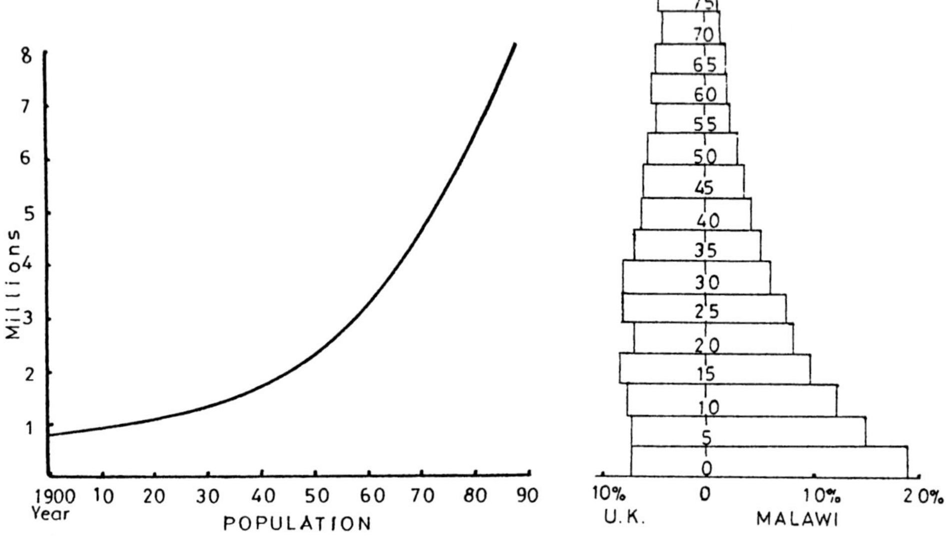

Malaŵi's population growth.

Comparison of % of population at different ages - Malaŵi and U.K.

CHILD HEALTH

"During a house to house visit among Christians in Ngoniland, we found that in one district, out of 230 children born to Church members, 180 had died. In another district, out of 79 born, 42 had died. Yet these districts would not be considered unhealthy. a great deal of this mortality is the result of ignorance and gross carelessness and might be prevented." (Dr.R. Laws 1903)

This was the first local report of the situation, and it is disturbing to reflect how long it was before it was possible to focus attention on these sorts of figures. 150 mothers were questioned by Dr.Mrs. Agnes Fraser in 1924 at Embangweni, and of the 611 children they had borne, 309 had died, (50% infant mortality rate). In 1932, Dr.Austin conducted an infant mortality survey in the Karonga district by questioning fathers. He found an under-6 death rate of over 40%.

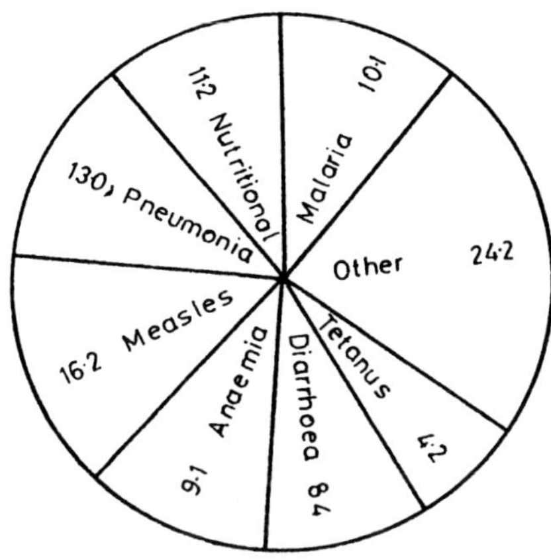

Causes of death in under 5's in hospital 1985 (%).

"One owes respect to the living; but to the dead one owes nothing but the truth."Voltaire

Today a third of all children never reach their 5th birthday, and many are under nourished or prone to disease. Since half the population of the country is under 15 years of age, the health of this half and their mothers is a major concern today. Even in 1940, the Annual Report stated:"Government Hospitals do little midwifery and Child Welfare." Mission hospitals started to run children's clinics in 1947.

Since Independence there has been considerable improvement. The first Child Specialist was appointed in 1964, Dr.Mrs.A. Borgstein from Holland, (she was the wife of the Chief Surgeon, and the mother of 7 sons, 6 of whom have qualified as doctors, and 4 of whom have worked in Malaŵi). The need for Children's specialists was indicated by a Mission report in 1973: "It is not unusual that a sick child has all at one and the same time, chronic malaria, bilharzia, hookworm, ascaris worms, pneumonia, and anaemia, all underlying kwashiorkor, a form of malnutrition. A crying miserable child, sometimes very swollen, sometimes very thin, with many areas of broken skin at all the joints, is a typical picture on admission."(Nchalo)

At this time there was an expansion in Under Fives clinics and many mothers received their Green Cards on which details of the child's weight and immunization were entered. The health of the child is closely related to the mother's health and the mother's burden is great. More than a quarter of all families have no male bread-winners, and much of the farming is done by women. The average family size is 7·6 children. The health of the child is also related to the mother's level of education. In 1977, 83% of

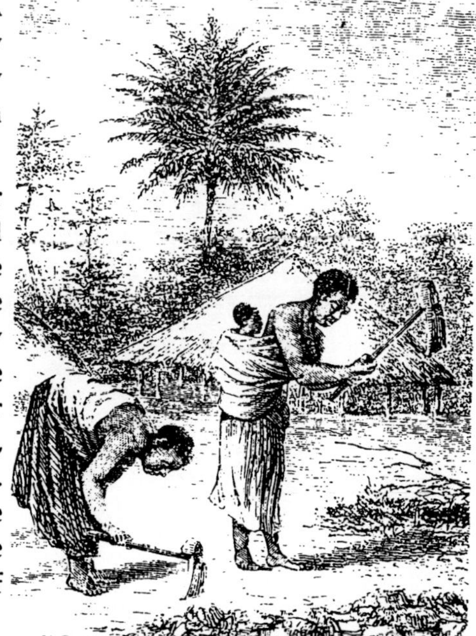

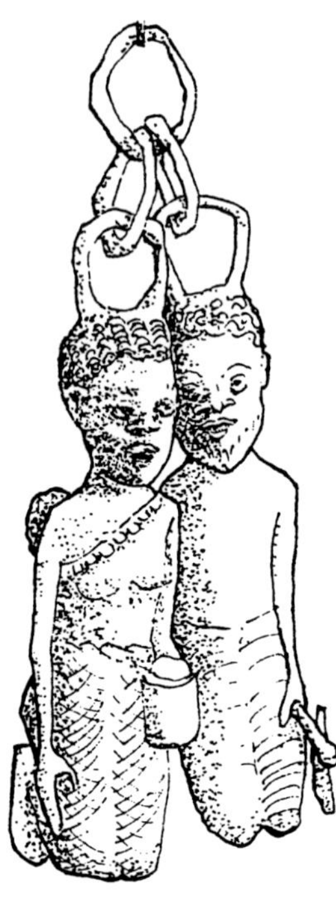

Local wood carving

women and 60% of men above 15 years were illiterate. There is a great desire for education, although less than one third of those who enrol at school stay for four years to reach basic literacy, because of financial difficulties. The success of so many development improvement measures in health, child spacing, Aids information, agricultural and small business matters, is related to levels of education. This is the vital step.

There is no doubt of the popularity of the under-fives children's clinics, mostly run by nurses and medical assistants. Today there is a very good coverage of the young population by the Extended Programme of Immunization against TB, Diphtheria, Polio, Measles, and Tetanus. By 1982, there were over a thousand under-fives clinics, well attended, and supervised today by an increasing number of Child Specialists.

FAMILY HEALTH IN THE 1990s

The rapidly increasing population in Malawi (it is estimated at over 9 million (1991) and at the present rate will double in 20 years), coupled with the new killer disease Aids, has changed the health emphasis in the family. Maintaining one sexual partner in a happy marriage has become a first priority to avoid Aids. Today it is important that the dignity of the instincts and emotions of both man and wife are respected. Modern methods of birth control are a means of improving the quality of sexual relations within marriage. As the survival of children depends on the happiness, health, and economic status of the mother, contraception has to be a feature of efforts to reduce infant mortality. Unplanned, unwanted, children are more likely to perish.

Methods of Contraception	
the hormonal pill	spermicidal foam
the intra-uterine loop	hormone implants
the condom or sheath	tubal ligation of the woman
depo provera injection	tubal ligation of the man
cervical cap (Dutch cap)	(vasectomy)

FUTURE HEALTH

It is appropriate to conclude with children, they are the future. Today, the great grandchildren of the individuals in the early chapters face new diseases and hazards to health. To our ancestors "Health for All" might have seemed a reasonable and even attainable goal. Today it is seen as more complex and we wonder how close our own great grandchildren may approach it. It is not the health of the individual alone that has to be considered, but also that of the community and ultimately of the planet. This state of health must be sustainable if future generations are not to suffer. This means conservation of scarce or non renewable resources like species of plants or animals, oil, soil, trees; control of pollution; sustainable increases in food production, education, employment, medicines, etc. to keep pace with population growth. It will mean a reduction in family size. The developed one fifth of the world with its stable population, uses far more energy, minerals, and water, than the developing world with its soaring population growth, and this equally needs to be redressed.

The long term outlook is daunting; however the example of our forebears gives inspiration and encouragement for this task.

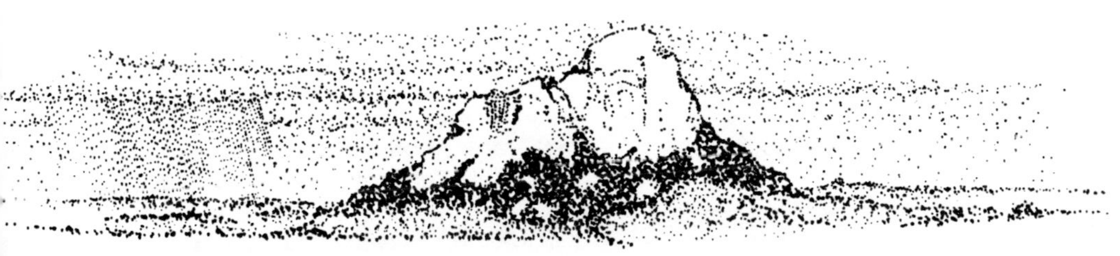

Hora Mountain

SOME COMPARATIVE DATA FOR THE 1980s

	U.S.A.	U.K	Sweden	Kenya	Tanzania	Malawi
GNP per head (1982) US$	13,160	9,960	14,040	390	280	230
Life expectancy at birth(1980)	75	74	77	57	47	47
Infant mortality rate*	11	11	7	77	98	151
Population per hospital bed (1980)	150	120	70	760	700	580
Population per physician (1980)	520	650	490	7,890	17,560	55,785**
Urban population % (1982)	78	91	88	15	13	8.5(1977)

* in first year of life per 1000 live births   **30,405 if Clinical Officers included

Sources: World Development Report, World Bank 1981, State of the World's Children UNICEF 1990, 1988 WHO Statistics.

Picture sources, some from books in the bibliography.

Page numbers given first: 5, 8, 11, 26, 43, 167, Livingstone's Journals; 15, 16, 111, Rowley; 1, 95 Faulkener; 4, Thomas Baines; 9, Kirk; 13, Anderson Morshead; 27, 40, Gelfand "Lakeside Pioneers"; 28, 29, 36, W.P. Livingstone; 38, Aurora; 44, Life and Work; 43, 137, Nyasaland Medical reports; 49, 120, Livingstonia News; 50, 52, Fotheringham; 53, 104, 105, 149, Society of Malawi Collection; 55, 126, Wellcome Library, London; 64, U.M.C.A. Reports; 71, 74, Elmslie; 72, Lovedale Press; 73, Campbell; 82, 83, Malamulo, Makwasa; 89, Frank Johnston; 91, Central African Medical Journal; 92, Zomba, Government Archives; 97, Harvey Goodwin ''Memoir of Bishop Mackenzie''; 110, 129, Dr.C. Blignaut; 115 Robert Koch Institute, reproduced in Health and Disease, Life series; 116, Johnston; 124 Moyo Magazine; 125, John Wilson; 140, D. Burkitt; 154 Federal Government Health Report; 157, MANA; 162 Gwen Gibbs; 163 Hans Gelderblom, Berlin; 23, 127,. Other illustrations, maps, and cover by M.S.K.

BIBLIOGRAPHY - Sources and further reading

Aurora, A Journal of Missionary News, (Livingstonia Mission Press 1897 - 1907).

Anderson Morshead,A.E.M. *The History of the Universities Mission to Central. Africa 1859-1909* (London, U.M.C.A. 1955).

Baker,C.A. *Johnston's Administration*, (Zomba; Government Press 1970).

Baker,Colin *Government Medical Services in Malawi, an Administrative History 1891-1974*, (typescript in the National Archives, Zomba).

Berry,W.T.C. *Before the Wind of Change* (England, Halesworth Press 1985).

Blantyre Church Nyasaland (Blantyre, Hetherwick Press 1926).

Blue Books, Annual Hospital Returns for the Protectorate of British Central Africa later Nyasaland.

Campbell,George H. *Lonely Warrior, William Koyi* (Blantyre,Claim 1975).

Central Africa, *Reports of the work of the UMCA* (London, U.M.C.A. from 1883 onwards).

Central African Planter (Zomba, Hynde and Stark 1895).

Cole King,P.A. *Cape Maclear* (Malaŵi Government 1968).

Cole King,P.A. *Lake Malawi Steamers* (Malawi Government 1971).

Colvin,Tom *Fathers and Founders of the Blantyre Synod* (Blantyre,CCAP 1976).

Cross,D.Kerr *Health in Africa*, (London,James Nisbet 1897).

Coupland,R. *Kirk on the Zambesi*, (Oxford, Oxford University Press 1928).

Daughters of Wisdom of the Shire Mission, historical report at Mlambe Hospital.

Dory,Electra *Leper Country* (Worcester, Trinity Press 1963).

Elmslie,W.A. *Among the Wild Angoni* (Edinburgh, Oliphant Anderson and Ferrier 1899).

Elton,J.F. *Travels and Researches among the Lakes and Mountains of East and Central Africa* (London, John Murray 1879).

Faulkner,Henry *Elephant Haunts*, (London, Hurst and Blackett 1868).

Federation of Rhodesia and Nyasaland, *Federal Government Health Reports 1952-63.*

Fotheringham, L.Monteith *Adventures in Nyassaland* (London 1891, reprinted in Malaŵi by M.A.P. 1987).

Gunther A. *Report on a collection of reptiles and fishes made by Dr. Kirk in the Zambesi Nyasa regions* (Proceedings of the Zoological Society of London 1864).

Geddie,John *The Lake Regions of Central Africa*, (London,T.Nelson 1898).

Gelfand,Michael *Livingstone the Doctor* (Oxford, Basil Blackwell 1957).

Gelfand,Michael *Lakeside Pioneers 1875-1920* (Oxford, Basil Blackwell 1964).

Gelfand,Michael *Rivers of Death in Africa* (Oxford, O.U.P. 1964).

Gelfand,Michael *Proud Record in Health Services in Rhodesia and Nyasaland* (Salisbury Rhodesia, Government Printer 1960).

Glemser,Bernard *The Long Safari* (London, The Bodley Head 1971).

Howson,P.J. *A Short History of Karonga* (Zomba, Government Press 1970).

Hine,J.E. Bishop *Days Gone By,* (London, John Murray 1924).

Jack,J.W. *Daybreak at Livingstonia,* (London, Oliphant et al. 1901).

Jeal,Tim *Livingstone,* (London, William Heinemann 1973, Penguin edition 1975).

Johnston,Sir Harry H. *British Central Africa,* (London, Methuen 1897).

Johnson,J. *Dr.Laws of Livingstonia,* (London, Partridge 1908).

Kirk,Sir John *Zambesi Journal and Letters 1858-63* (ed. R.Foskett Edinburgh 1965).

Kirk,Sir John *List of Mammalia met with in Zambesia,* (Proceedings of the Zoological Society, London 1864).

Laws Robert *Reminiscences of Livingstonia,* (Edinburgh, Oliver and Boyd 1934).

Life and Work in British Central Africa, (Blantyre Mission Reports from 1894).

Livingstone David *The Narrative of an Expedition to the Zambesi and its tributaries,* (London, John Murray 1865).

Livingstone,David *On Fever in the Zambesi,* (a note to Dr.M'William transmitted via the Admiralty, Lancet 1862).

Livingstone,David *The Last Journals,* (London, John Murray 1880).

Livingstone,W.P. *Laws of Livingstonia,* (London, Hodder and Stoughton 1921).

Livingstonia Mission of the Free Church of Scotland - Eleven Years' History and Appeal, (General Assembly of the Church of Scotland at Edinburgh in 1886).

Livingstonia News (Livingstonia Mission Press 1908-22).

Lugard,Lord F. D. *The Rise of our East African Empire,* (London, Blackwood 1893).

Maugham,R.C.F. *Africa as I have known it,* (London, John Murray 1929),

Manson's Tropical Diseases (19th edition Ballier Tindal, London 1987).

Meller,Charles J. *Fevers of the South East Coast of Africa,* (B. M. J., 25 Oct. 1862).

Meller,Charles J. *On the Fever of East Central Africa encountered by Livingstone's Zambesi Expedition,* (The Lancet for October 22nd and November 5th 1864).

Malaŵi Government, Annual Report of the Ministry of Health for 1964.

Malaŵi Statistical Year Book 1987 (Zomba, published by Malaŵi Government).

Medical Quarterly, Journal of the Malaŵi Medical Association 1980-91.

Moni Magazine for October 1983, and December 1989 (Blantyre, Montfort Press).

Morris,B *Medicines and Herbalism in Malaŵi,* (Soc. of Malaŵi J., Vol.42 No.2).

Mowschenson,Henry *Dr.H. Kamuzu Banda, President of the Republic of* Malaŵi, (Central African Journal of Medicine, August 1966).

Mponda Mission Diary 1889-1891 The White Fathers, Malaŵi.

Nyasaland Protectorate Annual Government Health and Sanitary Reports.

Pauw, Christoff Martin *Mission and Church in Malaŵi,* (Nkhoma CCAP 1980).

Praetorius, Pauline *Mission Hospitals in the Federation,* (Central African Medical Journal Vol.2 No.6, June 1956).

Principles and Practice of Tropical Medicine, (Napier, The Macmillan Co. , New York 1946).

Principles of Medicine in Africa, (ed E.H.O. Parry, O U P 1984).

Poole, Wordsworth Journals and Letters, (in the National Archives, and also edited by Michael Gelfand in the Central African Journal Medicine 1961).

Ransford, Oliver *Livingstone's Lake,* (London, John Murray 1966).

Retief, M.W. *William Murray of Nyasaland,* (translated from Afrikaans, South Africa, The Lovedale Press 1958).

Rowley, Henry *The Story of the Universities' Mission to Central Africa,* (London, Saunders Otley 1867).

Scott, Archibald Campbell *Journal of Livingstonia Mission 1891-95,* (Blantyre, Society of Malaŵi 1986).

Sim, Arthur Fraser *Life and Letters,* (London, U.M.C.A. 1896).

Simpkin, Alice *Nursing in Nyasaland,* (London, U.M.C.A. 1925).

Stewart, Dr.J. *The Zambesi Journal 1862-3,* (London, Chatto and Windus 1865).

Stewart, James *From Nyassa to Tanganyika,* (Blantyre, Central Africana 1989).

Smit, J.J.M. The *role of the Dutch Reformed Church Mission in the development of Nursing in Nyasaland from 1860-1927,* (Ph.D. thesis Stellensbosch Univ. for 1986).

UMCA Letters at Rhodes House, Oxford.

UNICEF *The situation of Children and Women in Malaŵi,* (Lilongwe 1987).

UNICEF *The Child and the Nation,* (1989). *The State of the World's Children* (1990).

University of Malaŵi *Workshop of Household Food and Security and Nutrition,* (Zomba, Centre for Social Research 1988).

Wallis, J.P.R. *The Zambesi Expedition of David Livingstone,* (London, Chatto and Windus 1956).

Watson, W.H. *Eheu Fugaces Labuntur Anni* (Central African Journal of Medicine, March 1955).

Yarnton Mills, Dora S. *What we do in Nyasaland,* (London, U.M.C.A. 1911).

Yearbook and Guide of Rhodesias and Nyasaland 1963, (Rhodesian Pub. Ltd).

Young, E.D. *The Search after Livingstone,* (London, John Murray 1868; facsimile Blantyre, Society of Malaŵi and Royal Geographical Society 1984).

Young, E.D. *Nyassa, A Journal of Adventures,* (London, John Murray 1877; facsimile Blantyre Rotary Club 1984).

WHO *Statistics Annual* 1988.

CHRONOLOGY OF SOME IMPORTANT EVENTS

1857	Livingstone's Senate House Speech. Cambridge.
1859	Livingstone reaches Lake Malaŵi.
1861	U.M.C.A. Mission at Magomero, Dr.Dickinson first resident doctor.
1863	U.M.C.A. leave.
1866	*Pasteur describes bacteria spoiling wine in France.*
1867	*Lister describes antisepsis in Scotland.*
1874	*Hansen (Norway) describes first bacterial cause of human disease – leprosy.*
1875	Laws and Young found Livingstonia at Cape Maclear and circumnavigate the Lake.Thousands of slaves crossing the country .
1876	Blantyre founded by Scottish missionaries. Arrival of Lovedale evangelists, Koyi, Dr.Stewart, Dr.Black at Cape Maclear.
	First chloroform case in Central Africa by Dr. Laws at Cape Maclear.
1878	Coffee planted.
	Laws and Koyi meet Ngoni Chief Chikusi.
	Livingstone Central African Co.Ltd. formed.
	Margaret Gray marries Robert Laws at Blantyre Church.
1879	Laws and Koyi meet Ngoni Chief M'mbelwa. U.M.C.A. return.
1880	*Laveran (Algeria) shows Malaria parasites in blood.*
1881	Dr.Laws moves Livingstonia to Bandawe from Cape Maclear.
1882	Koyi opens mission at Njuyu to Chief M'mbelwa's Ngoni.
	Koch (Germany) describes TB bacillus.
	Pasteur (France) demonstrates immunity against some diseases.
1883	Captain Foote first British Consul.
1884	Dr.Kerr Cross opens Mwiniwanda Mission.
	A.L.C. store at Karonga (Fotheringham).
	Domasi Mission opens.
	Dr.Elmslie starts medical work at Njuyu Village.
1885	*Treaty of Berlin (partition of Africa).*
1887	Slave Wars at Karonga.
	Dr.Laws and Ngoni Chief M'mbelwa meet.
	Dr.Bowie arrives at Blantyre.
1888	Harry Johnston appointed British Consul.
	Foundation of St. Michael's Church, Clement Scott.

1889   Andrew Murray starts Dutch Reformed Mission at Mvera.

Temporary peace with slaver Mlozi at Karonga.

Dr.Hine first doctor at Likoma Island UMCA.

1890   British Government ultimatum, Portuguese leave Shire Valley.

Rinderpest (cattle) epidemic.

Harry Johnston requests gunboats for the Lake.

Dr.George Steele comes to Njuyu.

Dr.Affleck Scott goes to Blantyre then Domasi.

Smallpox epidemic.

1891   Cecil Rhodes promises Johnston aid for British Central Africa (British territories north of the Zambesi).

Sikh soldiers and Indian traders arrive. Forts built.

Dr.Sorabji Boyce first Government doctor. Smallpox epidemic.

Behring (Germany) develops diphtheria anti-toxin.

1892   Zambezi Industrial Mission arrive. Ngoni raids on the Nkonde.

Government campaigns against Yao chiefs. Jiggers reaches the Lake.

1894   Tanganyika removed from Johnston's control.

Dr.Laws moves Livingstonia to Khondowe.

Telegraph Salisbury/Blantyre started.

Dr.George Prentice comes to Bandawe.

1895   Administration extended over all Nyasaland except to the Northern Ngoni people.

Dr.Wordsworth Poole arrives at Zomba.

Further campaigns against the Yao Chiefs in the South.

Mlozi defeated and hanged at Karonga.

Rontgen (Germany) discovers X rays.

1896   African population estimated at 1 million.

Increased use of cash (as opposed to cloth) payment.

Cape Maclear Mission handed over to the DRC.

Locust plague at Khondowe. Rinderpest epidemic.

H.Johnston leaves for Tunis. Post office runners Blantyre to Zomba night mail.

Dr.Eykman (Dutch E. I.) demonstrated vitamin deficiency in chickens.

1897   Blantyre European Hospital opened.

1898   Hut tax levied in North Nyasa.

	Bicycle in Blantyre.

Bicycle in Blantyre.

Telegraph link Europe - Blantyre - Livingstonia.

Ross (India) demonstrates malaria/mosquito link.

1899   Dr.Howard arrives at Likoma Island. Smallpox epidemic.

Aspirin first synthesized.

1900   First General Conference of Missionaries at Blantyre (Dr.Elmslie as chairman). Smallpox epidemic.

S.African General Mission at Lulwe.

1901   Chauncy Maples assembled at Mponda's.

Catholic Mission at Nzama.

Likoma Hospital opened.

1902   Decision to build Chiromo/Blantyre Railway. Seventh Day Adventists at Makwasa.

UMCA hospital at Nkhota Kota (Miss K. Mintner).

Dr.J.B.Davey (Government) arrives.

1903   Level of Lake lowest in living memory.

Livingstone Hospital, Zomba, opened by Livingstone's daughter, Mrs.A.L.Bruce

Famine at Port Herald.

WENELA (Witwatersrand Native Labour Association) set up 3-4,000 Nyasaland workers per year go to S.Africa, labour regulations regarding food and health

1904   Ngoni agree to be a part of Nyasaland. Blind school at Nkhota Kota. 7 doctors in Government service.

Systematic smallpox vaccination.

1905   Telephone lines reach Livingstonia Dr.Stannus arrives.

Medical Assistant training courses in Blantyre.

1907   Government Sleeping Sickness post at Karonga.

Ehrlich (Germany) discovers Salvarsan.

British Central Africa renamed Nyasaland.

1908   First train Port Herald/Blantyre.

First Barium meal (Germany).

1909   Interest in hookworm.

1910   Lake at low level.

1911   David Gordon Memorial Hospital opened at Livingstonia. Dr.Stannus described pellagra at Zomba.

Mwabvi ordeal declared illegal. Smallpox.

1914 *First World War*. Battle at Karonga after the Germans cross the Songwe River.

7 of 11 government doctors recruited to military duties. Medical Assistant training at Likoma.

1915 Chilembwe Rising.

1916 Plague in North Nyasaland.

1918 *First World War ends.*

Antimony tartrate injection for bilharzia.

Influenza pandemic (5,000 deaths in Lilongwe).

1920 *Carbon tetrachloride first used against hookworm U.S.A.*

Banting and Best (Canada) extract insulin.

1922 Drought and famine 2,300 tons of food distributed.

1925 Polio epidemic.

Dr.Malekebu, first Nyasaland doctor returns from U.S.A.

1927 First X-ray machine at Livingstonia.

1928 Dr.Laws departs after 53 years of service.

Fleming (Britain) describes penicillin.

1930 Smallpox. Hookworm campaigns.

Nightsoil collections in Blantyre and Zomba. Blantyre, piped water from Hynde Dam.

1932 Lilongwe piped water from river.

1937 Meningitis epidemic.

Domagck (Germany) releases first sulphonamide.

1938 Nutritional surveys.

1939 *Second World War*, many Malawians in King's African Rifles serve overseas.

1941 *Florey and Chain (Britain) extract penicillin for use in patients.*

1944 *Streptomycin discovered by Waksman (U.S.A.).*

1945 *End of Second World War.*

DDT and Gammexane first non-toxic effective insecticides become more widely available.

1947 Famine in South.

1949 Smallpox.

1950 Zomba Mental Hospital upgraded.

1951   Sulphones used for leprosy and streptomycin for TB used in Nyasaland.

1952   *Tetracycline discovered.*

1953   Federation of Rhodesia and Nyasaland,increase in healthfunding.

1954   Last cases of yaws.

Polio epidemic.

Salk Polio Vaccines used in U.S.A.

1957   *Sabin oral Polio vaccine used in U.S.A.*

1958   Dr H. Kamuzu Banda returns to Nyasaland.

The Queen Mother opened the Queen Elizabeth Hospital, Blantyre.

1959   Anti Federation disturbances.

1960   Malaŵians sent abroad for nursing training. Smallpox.

Oral Polio Vaccine in the country.

1963   Piped water from Shire River for Blantyre.

Many expatriate doctors leave as Federation breaks up. Three Malaŵian doctors return.

1964   Malaŵian Independence.

Medical Association of Malaŵi formed.

1965   PHAM Private Hospital Association of Malaŵi formed.

National School of Nursing opens. LEPRA set up in Malaŵi.

1971   Last cases of smallpox in Malaŵi.

1973   Cholera enters S. Malaŵi.

1977   *Last case of smallpox in the world (Somalia).*

1979   Save the Children Fund Stop Polio vaccination campaign.

1980   Malaŵi Against Polio, funding from Rotary International.

1981   *Aids first recorded (U.S.A.).*

1982   Rifampicin used in leprosy.

1983   *Aids virus isolated.*

1984   Aids first confirmed in Malaŵi.

1986   20 Malaŵians each year go to U.K. for next for five years medical training, returning to complete final year in new Medical College of Malaŵi.

1991   College of Medicine opens.

INDEX

THE STORY OF AIDS IN MALAWI

AIDS has come to dominate the pathology and sociology of Malawi and has overtaken malaria as the major cause of death. Life expectancy has fallen from 47 years in 1984 to 36 years today. There are about 84,000 new orphans each year.

Present knowledge of Acquired Immune Deficiency Disease
In 1981 clinical AIDS was first diagnosed amongst homosexuals in America and by 1983 the Human Immune-deficiency Virus was identified. Tests to diagnose the disease have improved over the years. They rely on detecting antibodies to the virus, although this does not happen until a few months after infection (the 'window' period). In Malawi today a finger prick test produces a result within five minutes. Tests for the actual virus are complex but can be done at a few centres.

HIV is a retro-virus made from RNA, a minute particle wrapped in a capsule. It targets and enters certain cells, especially blood CD4 lymphocytes responsible for immunity. It imprints itself on the DNA of the nucleus, forcing it to make millions more copies, and so producing high levels of circulating HIV in the body fluids - blood, semen, vaginal secretions and breast milk.

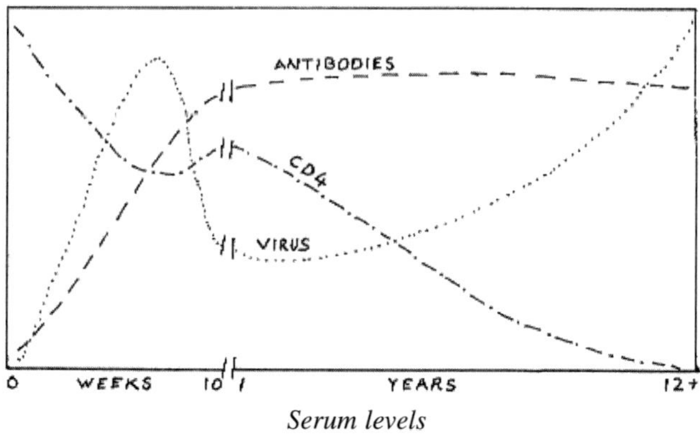

Serum levels

A few weeks after HIV-infection, there may be a 'flu like illness and then the patient becomes asymptomatic. The viral load slowly increases and the CD4 cells are gradually destroyed, until at a varying period of time after infection, from months to ten years, the level of immunity drops and opportunistic infections occur. Typically HIV patients are then prone especially to TB and also to shingles, dermatitis, diarrhoea, bacterial infections, herpes, oral and vaginal thrush, pneumonia, and Kaposi's Sarcoma. Clinical diagnosis of AIDS can be made at this time. The disease worsens and the patient dies.

Anti-Retro Viral drugs inhibit the enzymes involved in HIV replication and make viral load undetectable. But they do not eliminate the HIV-imprint on the DNA in the host cell. Once infected, a victim can never get rid of this virus. If the ARV drugs are not taken regularly, the virus is produced again and more serious drug resistance may develop. In Malawi, ARV treatment is started at WHO clinical Stage 3 or Stage 4 of the disease when the CD count is falling. Three drugs are combined in a tablet, to be taken twice daily.

Story of the AIDS Pandemic in Malawi
The precursor of HIV crossed species from a chimpanzee to a human in Cameroon around 1929, probably by close contact with blood. AIDS was not recognized as a clinical disease in Malawi until 1985.

Analysis of dried blood on filter paper samples taken and stored from 44,000 people during a leprosy survey in Karonga in the early 1980s offers historic and most interesting insight into the arrival of this virus in Malawi. Multiple introductions of the HIV-1 subtypes A and D viruses in 1981-2 were not very infectious. But once HIV-1 subtype C, arrived in 1983, it spread rapidly. The explosive growth of subtype C cluster probably arose from a single introduction in or before 1983.

We know that in Karonga, adult HIV-prevalence rose from 0.1% in 1981, to 2% by 1989. Soon HIV-1C prevailed across Malawi. Only in 1985 were the first clinical cases of 'full blown AIDS' diagnosed in Blantyre and Lilongwe. Clinicians were seeing increasing numbers of patients with enlarged lymph nodes and aggressive Kaposi's Sarcoma. Soon this became a major outbreak.

The course of this heterosexually transmitted disease in Malawi is an example of exponential, rapidly increasing growth. However this spreading infection may also indicate that the genes of the HIV-1C virus found a compatible genetic host in the local population. In the Southern Africa region HIV-1C causes 90% of AIDS infections. (HIV-1B spread by homosexuals and drug abusers prevailed in Europe and America).

<table>
<tr><td colspan="6">HIV-prevalence in women at the free Ante-Natal Clinic at Queen Elizabeth Hospital Blantyre</td></tr>
<tr><td>1985</td><td>2%</td><td>1990</td><td>22%</td><td>1994</td><td>32%</td></tr>
<tr><td>1986</td><td>3%</td><td>1991</td><td>26%</td><td>1995</td><td>33%</td></tr>
<tr><td>1987</td><td>8%</td><td>1992</td><td>27%</td><td>1996</td><td>35%</td></tr>
<tr><td>1988</td><td>19%</td><td>1993</td><td>30%</td><td>1997</td><td>37%</td></tr>
</table>

It is estimated that 98% of HIV transmission in Malawi is by unprotected sexual intercourse. The risk of catching AIDS by clinical contact seems to be low. An interesting survey of AIDS mortality amongst hundreds of teachers and health care workers in urban Malawi, surprisingly found that more teachers (2.3%) than health care workers (2%) had died after 'chronic illness' in 1999.

HIV is killing all strands of our people, politicians, doctors, nurses, clergy, teachers and police, just to mention a few.....it costs government about K80,000 a year to keep one student in our institutions of higher learning for 4-5 years of training. It is sobering to note that at the current rate of life expectancy, most of them will serve only ten years before they die of AIDS. (Newspaper article by a Malawian doctor in 2001)

Malnutrition does not increase the risk of catching HIV, but it does cause immune impairment, contributing to a more rapid progression to full blown AIDS.

Children

About half the children born to HIV-mothers die of AIDS. In 28% of babies, intra-uterine transmission of the HIV-virus occurs. Probably the remaining 22% of children acquire the virus from breast feeding. Since 2004, neviraprin has been given to HIV-mothers before delivery to lower the risk of HIV-transmission; but viral resistance to this drug is now occurring in South Africa.

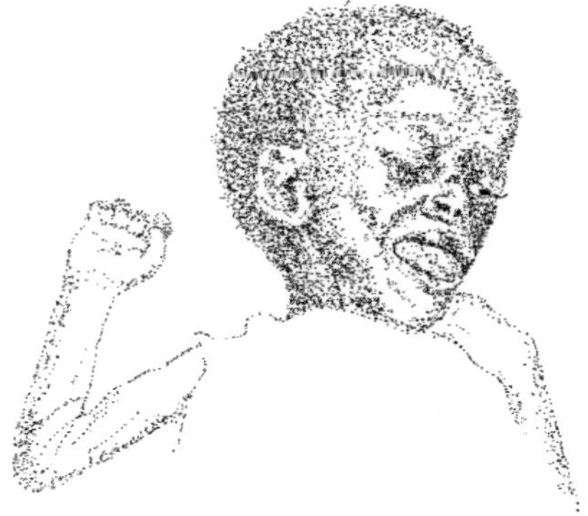

Failure To Thrive - AIDS

Efficient family planning services targeting AIDS-mothers avert more HIV-infected births than neviraprin programmes. It is now common to see grandmas sitting by half the sick children in the ward, because mother has already died.

Women

The U.N. observed that in Africa AIDS has a woman's face. This typical face is wasted with a rash, swollen glands, thinning hair, and premature ageing.

The Karonga blood samples collected 1980-89 showed HIV-prevalence was highest among persons with good education, with better jobs, and with better housing. This social fact has been confirmed in subsequent studies in Malawi. Analysis of 1995 data from Blantyre pregnant mothers showed that a woman whose husband had been more than 8 years at school was twice as likely to be HIV- positive than a lady with a less educated husband. The 1996 Lilongwe Survey reported the highest HIV rates in women whose partners were professionals, skilled workers or in the Military, including Police. High rates were found in professional and skilled women. Educated women were three times more likely to be HIV-positive than illiterate women.

In 1998 World Bank reported that the HIV-infection rate amongst Blantyre pregnant women in the 25-29 year age group was 44%. And a 1999/2000 survey of all patients in Blantyre hospital wards in two weeks showed that 'being female, better educated, and aged 21-29 is to be at highest risk of testing positive for HIV.'

It is sad but true that educated ladies are no less likely to risk catching AIDS than their illiterate sisters. Among teenagers, HIV-prevalence rates are six time higher for girls than for boys. Women are biologically more vulnerable to this disease. Of Malawian adults infected with HIV, 59% are female. All statistics must be viewed with caution in Africa, but these estimates suggest the scale of the problem.

Pregnancy
Although pregnant mothers at antenatal clinics have been HIV-tested anonymously for two decades in Malawi, there has been little enquiry into their survival. There have not been public warnings that women carrying the HIV-virus face grave perils in childbearing.

A woman's immunity is lowered during pregnancy to ensure the mother's body does not reject the foetus, which is a genetically foreign body. This means the chances of an HIV-mother developing full blown AIDS during or after pregnancy are much higher than without going through the pregnancy. It also has to be considered that there is a 35% chance of the mother transmitting HIV to the baby. (Newspaper report from a Malawian doctor at the College of Medicine.)

This is a strong case for all HIV-positive expectant mothers to be offered termination of pregnancy. Medical or surgical abortion could allow an HIV-positive woman to survive for many years longer to look after her other children.

HIV-mothers often become severely anaemic and wasted. In Malawi increasing numbers of HIV-women die during pregnancy and childbirth or within six weeks afterwards. These are classified as 'maternal deaths', usually caused by severe HIV-anaemia which does not improve with a blood transfusion, ruptured uterus, or sepsis which does not respond to antibiotics. A terrible way to die.

One in seven Malawian women now has a lifetime chance of dying of pregnancy related causes - the 1.2% official maternal death rate is the third highest in the world. But the real maternal death rate is probably greater. Midwives note that some mothers are 'going downhill' at the post-natal appointment six weeks after delivery, and die within six months of childbirth. The number of children orphaned by AIDS is estimated in 2006 to be a million, or 20% of all children in Malawi.

Survival with AIDS
Some AIDS victims develop full blown AIDS within a year or two of HIV infection. But a few are infected for many years with low viral loads and competent immune systems. At Karonga in 2001, a retrospective survey of nearly 4,000 AIDS victims showed they had a median survival time of eight years; 70% alive after five years, and 36% surviving to ten years. But all had died within fourteen years.
With plagues in the past, a human immunity has developed after several generations. Today some individuals live with HIV for years before succumbing to it - perhaps due to genetic factors. Some day vaccines may be developed. HIV might diminish in virulence. Society may eventually change, with stricter controls on behaviour.

There are so many deaths in our village now that work in the fields is jeopardized. There have been five funerals this week, and on each day no weeding was allowed by custom. (2002)

The Global Fund - treatment and preventive efforts
From 1999, ARV treatment was available at the Lighthouse clinic in Lilongwe and other private clinics. Firms were asked to pay for ARV drugs by their employees. By 2001 the UN Global Fund, supported by international donor governments like USA, UK, other G8 and non G8 countries and the World Bank, aimed to reduce AIDS mortality, treat patients, prevent new HIV-infections, and support orphan care. It donated US $190 million as a five year budget to the Malawi National AIDS

Commission in 2003. This was a huge sum to dispense through chosen NGOs - sometimes to uneducated village groups trying to look after orphans. Submitting proposals and accounting were inevitably a problem.

Almost everybody, including children, in this district is very well informed about AIDS and how it is spread, but this has not caused behaviour change. Knowledge about HIV cannot be equated with avoiding it, even though most families have seen relatives die. The evidence from other delegates at the Blantye AIDS conference corroborated this. (Ekwendeni Survey in 2001)

People who know they have AIDS now avoid coming clinics where they will be HIV-tested, this includes ante-natal clinics (Nurse 2005)

Huge funds have been spent on 'Behaviour Change' propaganda in schools, youth clubs, and the media. The ABC advice of 'Abstinence, Be faithful, and Condom use' has failed to limit the spread of HIV. Ideas of 'female empowerment' have not inspired chastity or matrimonial joy in Malawi. Millions of condoms have been distributed - to men at roadside bars by the EU, to youths at school by NGOs, and to prostitutes by UNDP - which also promoted a prostitutes' football team in Lilongwe in 2006. This has not constrained the HIV epidemic.

Shortage of health staff is a major obstacle. Community groups are trained in home-based care for HIV victims. Numerous NGOs and charities receive funding for orphan care and village income generating projects like maize mills. Grants are made to promote 'positive living' by people living with AIDS. Voluntary Counselling and Testing (VCT) clinics have been opened in 239 approved sites with public advice to know one's HIV-status.

By late 2005, sixty ART clinics had opened dispensing ARV drugs costing US$ 20 per month per client to 28,000 patients. While at the same time some hospitals were short of sutures, plaster of paris, cheap praziquantel to cure thousands with bilharzia, and quinine tablets to cure malaria. Already gravely

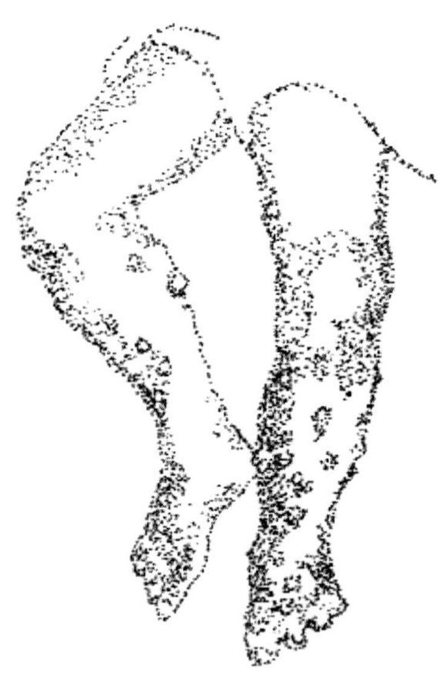

Kaposi's Sarcoma

understaffed, they had to cope with the extra burden of operating ART clinics for hundreds more patients each month.

Many Malawian HIV patients thrive on these drugs and return to work. But 25% die within three months, others die after taking ARVs for one year, and many default. Some can only manage light work. Common side effects of these drugs are pains in the legs and feet, rashes, headaches, vomiting, dizziness, diarrhoea, and jaundice.
Sometimes 'virological treatment failure' occurs during the course of ART with the viral load increasing - an ominous sign. The numbers of patients with viral resistance could also increase exponentially. A detectable viral load in 9% of patients was found at one city ART clinic in the first year. Eventually the virus will mutate to be resistant to these ARV drugs, resulting perhaps in a greater human tragedy.

The very expensive second line drugs are not freely available and require intensive supervision. Patients on ART have to come to the clinic every month for a check-up and renewed supplies of pills. This is only possible for those who live near a clinic, or who have money for transport. If they are weak they cannot make the journey.

ART clients are advised to abstain from unprotected sexual intercourse because an infected partner may increase his/her own viral load and mutations with other subtypes, leading to health deterioration and full blown AIDS.

Of the 960 AIDS clients I have counselled, about two thirds tell me they have currently more than three sexual partners - this is from my risk assessment forms. (AIDS counsellor)
The tales HIV clients tell us show they have taken little notice of the careful advice we gave them at the start of the ARV treatment programme. Many are problem people in bad matrimonial situations, polygamous marriages, divorced, open marriages, single mothers, lone males etc. They have several sexual partners and this is their lifestyle.... which they resume when they feel stronger with ARVs. I see no end to the spread of AIDS now. (ART clinician)

Treatment of HIV-infected children has recently started with splitting the tablets, but there are many problems in treating children.

Planners of ART programmes have done well, but have foreseen a fearsome task ahead. In crowded government hospitals the number of the HIV clients may double yearly, but only a fraction have access. There is no guarantee that the Global Fund can expand and continue indefinitely. It is secure only until 2008. Meanwhile new HIV-infections are steadily increasing.

Cultural Customs in Malawi

Various initiation rituals may spread HIV. Girl initiates are taught in songs and dances to be sexually willing. On the final night, a girl left alone in a hut is raped by an old man, called 'Fisi', meaning a hyena.
During male initiation, a dance is performed in the moonlight with drums beating and hand clapping; ululating women add to the melancholy of the song. Boys are taken away to a hut in the bush. One razor is used to cut the foreskins of several boys and they suffer much pain. For a week they eat relish without salt or oils and this has a magic effect. When the wounds heal, they have become men and must prove their manhood in promiscuous sex. (University student)

Ritual circumcision has not protected communities from AIDS; districts with these rituals have high rates of HIV. One project tried to persuade villagers to do away with these customs, described by the National AIDS Commission as lethal cultural beliefs.

Polygamy prevails in the patrilocal culture of North Malawi where each wife lives in her house in the husband's village: 'polygamous wives have other sexual partners, because one husband cannot satisfy several women.'(Nurse) In Chikamwini marriages customary in South Malawi, the husband goes to live at his wife's home and said 'because I am Mkamwini I am allowed to have other partners, and some of my lovers are my wife's relatives; I am free to date other women.'(Newspaper report)

Polygamists and their wives, dying of AIDS, now fill hospital wards. Malawi has no universal monogamous marriage laws in 2007, although some chiefs say polygamy should be abolished.

Many patients have resorted to traditional medicines from sing'angas, because they think illness is caused by witchcraft.

In 1996 a new sorcery cure for AIDS attracted huge crowds. Thousands of people from all corners of Malawi have been swarming to little known Chikanama village to drink a drug believed to cure AIDS. This was produced by the vision of old Mr. Chisupe. He dreamed of this purifying herbal potion 'mchape' made from the bark of a local tree. Such huge crowds came to drink his' mchape'that the village became a sanitation risk and government had to bring in water bowsers. Eventually the government pathologist announced that clients who had drunk Mr. Chisupe's 'mchape' continued to be HIV-positive and many then died. Mr. Chisupe was not deterred and argued that AIDS patients also die in hospitals despite modern medicines. (Newspaper rerport)

Human Rights, Denial and its results

Politicians initially concealed and denied the epidemic. In the 1980s President Banda's government was reluctant to admit to this rapidly spreading, new disease. Even by 1988, the Government pathologist was not allowed to give Malawian HIV-statistics to the World Health Organization. This was not the only form of dangerous political denial of the AIDS epidemic.

> *We are not facing the HIV problem, we have our heads in the sand. (Malawian professor)*

Pressurized by vociferous liberal and homosexual lobbies, United Nations politicians decreed in 1983 that everyone in the world must have the right <u>not</u> to bc HIV-tested - unless he/she consents to it. Thus foreign lawyers had a part in ensuring that the sexually transmitted HIV-1C which threatened the whole normal adult population and unborn children in Central Africa, remained a hidden danger.

The HIV-1B prevalent in USA and Europe was only transmitted easily by anal sex and blood injections; so the general hetero-sexual population and pregnant mothers are not so much at risk. Homosexual morality has no responsibility for pregnant mothers and future generations.

If AIDS had been initially managed as a deadly infection like SARS, Bird Flu, or leprosy, infected persons could possibly have been identified and the speed of the disease slowed down. But the long incubation period of the disease would not have allowed this. HIV-carriers are protected by UN human rights, and voluntary consent is required before HIV-testing.

Yet although they can endanger others, HIV-carriers must not be stigmatized. Under this protective cloak HIV-1C has spread to millions in Africa, with suffering worse then the holocaust. Did lawyers have a right to interfere with clinical medicine? The medical profession shares the blame by not insisting on a scientific approach. The value of surveys for other diseases is undermined if an HIV-test for every patient is not included. It has always been acceptable to test routinely for TB and syphilis as part a pre-employment medical examination, but not apparently for this more serious disease - HIV.

The counselling required by UNAIDS protocols both before and after HIV-testing takes far too long, so clinicians in overcrowded hospitals would often not have time to do an AIDS test on a sick patient. HIV-testing only with the patient's informed consent has also blindfolded physicians. Diagnosis in hospitals has often been reduced to intuition and the scientific basis of medicine flawed. For instance, it is often assumed that a patient not responding to treatment has AIDS, and so the diagnosis of a curable diseases like Sleeping Sickness is missed - and the chance to cure it. But diagnostic testing without asking for consent is now becoming more acceptable in 2007.

HIV-positive people are advised to shun contact with contagious diseases. They should avoid staying in hospital because of the risks of infection. This is a reason for HIV-testing all patients. HIV-positive health staff taking ARVs face similar perils in doing their job.

As the HIV-virus suppresses immunity, risks of surgical procedures may be increased and post-operative infection more common. If a surgeon is to be able to assess truthfully the risks of doing an operation, a routine HIV-test, like other routine blood tests, should be carried out on all surgical patients.

We believe there has been too much muddled thinking about AIDS in the rich world, produced by various pressure groups. Although compassion for HIV victims and their treatment is very important, the economic consequences of this epidemic must be faced. In Malawi, agriculture, business, public services, and the civil service are severely undermined by AIDS. Efficiency is jeopardized. An annual HIV-attrition rate of 2.3% amongst civil servants, health staff, teachers, water engineers, and policemen was quoted by UNDP in 2002.

The mandatory HIV-test for boys aspiring to become priests is not discriminatory but aims at identifying healthy people who can ably carry out pastoral work. (Episcopal Conference of Malawi 2003)

Some Christian schools have suggested bursaries for pupils who remain HIV-negative, but foreign donors threatened to withdraw support. (Newspaper report)

Teachers have died faster than they can be replaced, nurses, clinical officers, and doctors have died in large numbers - of the 20 doctors in the first graduating year at the College of Medicine, only eleven were alive a few years later (not all died of AIDS). A World Bank report to the Nairobi AIDS conference in 2003 predicted that up to half the professional workforce in Malawi would die of AIDS by 2005, with teachers, nurses and doctors being especially badly hit. More than half of ESCOM's staff needed extra health care in 2006.

Students have come to our country for expensive courses only to sicken and even die before graduating. We are not allowed to HIV-test before recruiting students for training, but if Malawians decided it was in the country's best interest, we would support it. (Donor Government diplomat)

The sad fact must be faced that training students who are already HIV-positive is not cost effective in Malawi; it is 'incapacity building', even when ARV drugs are available. It may deprive patients, children, and society of the greatly needed skills and services they would have had if a fit person had been trained. Yet compulsory testing has been forbidden by the rich world.

The prime time for catching the virus is 15-24 years. If only HIV-negative students were admitted to further education and training, this might result in behaviour change. The fear of testing HIV-positive would give young people an immediate incentive to avoid risky behaviour. This problem should be debated in Malawi and not dictated by lobbies from very different economic, cultural, and disease situations on the other side of the world.

MEDICINE AND DISEASE IN MALAWI 1992-2007

Since the publication of this book fifteen years ago, some medicine and disease patterns have changed. AIDS has come to dominate the pathology and sociology of the country.

In 1992, after donor pressure and rioting in Blantyre with deaths and hospital admissions for gunshot wounds, the autocratic Life President, Dr. Kamuzu Banda, sanctioned a referendum. Two years later came a fragile democracy. There is now more freedom of speech but no freedom from poverty. 60% of the population are below the poverty line, living on less than $2 per day. Malawi remains among the 10 poorest countries in the world with a per capita GDP of $600 per year. (UK $31.400)

In the early nineties the Mozambique civil war was drawing to a close and a million refugees in Malawi returned home. There were also droughts, and associated cholera, dysentery, and meningitis epidemics. The United Nations High Commission for Refugees provided extra funds for hospitals near the camps. New operating theatres were built in Blantyre to help with the refugee referrals, including battle casualties.

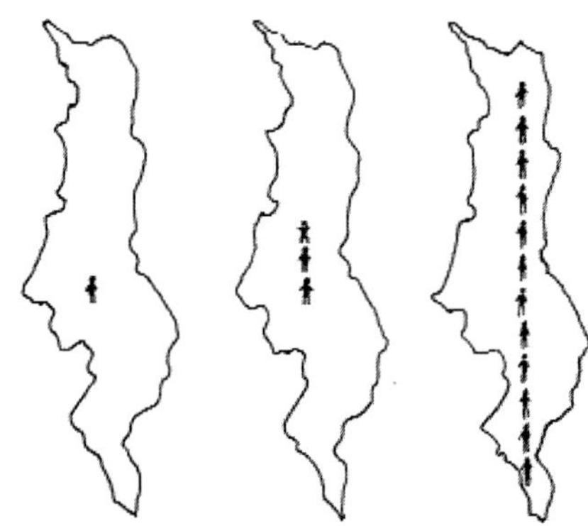

Population in 1900, 1950, 2005
Each figure = 1 million

Like the rest of the continent, Malawi is becoming poorer and more aid dependent, largely due to the population growth; it doubles every 20 years and has now reached 13 million. Malnutrition is ever present, food production and fish catches per head decline, and severe famine in 2002 caused several thousand deaths, the worst in living memory.

Medicine

The disease burden increases and the health services are hard pressed to cope. 60% of deaths are from infectious diseases alone, 20% from maternal, peri-natal, and nutritional conditions. In the rich world this total figure is 5%.

Two out of five babies die before the age of ten years. HIV has overtaken malaria as a major cause of death. Life expectancy has fallen from 47 years in 1988 to 36 in 2006, although most statistics from Africa must be accepted with caution.

Most of the sick go to the free Government services, and are young. Funding for these hospitals had been steadily falling. AIDS, emigration, and the rising numbers of NGOs has taken staff away from the overcrowded wards. In 2002, 90 out of 108 qualifying nurses went to the UK. Workshops and the more recent ART clinics regularly take staff away from sick patients. The nurse establishment in most hospitals is 40% unfilled. Rural Health Centres are short staffed or closed.

However in very recent years there are some signs of improvement. Debt relief in 2006 freed more funds for health and education. Considerable donor funds (from UK, Norway, Sweden, World Bank. and the Global Fund) have improved health staff take home pay. But a young doctor in 2006 only has $321 per month, after tax, to pay for rent, services and living expenses.

The total number of doctors in government service, many expatriates included, in 1999 was 103, with another 53 in Mission hospitals and a few more in private clinics. The College of Medicine opened in 1991 and produced about 20 doctors a year, recently the number in training has doubled. It was hoped that by now most of the District Hospitals would have one. But in 2006, only 13 of the 27 Government District Hospitals had Malawian doctors. The Ministry only manages to retain a few, Some stay on in Central hospitals or in better paid mission hospitals, or join research projects, go into private practice, join NGOs, emigrate, or have died. There are very few specialists in the country.

Human Resources in 2006, Govt and Mission

Cadre	Number in post	Vacancies	% in post
Physicians	*130*	*294*	*32%*
Nurses	*4717*	*3723*	*56%*
Clinical Officers	*942*	*463*	*67%*
Medical Assistants	*718*	*782*	*48%*
Laboratory technicians	*251*	*256*	*50%*
Pharmo techs	*93*	*192*	*50%*
Environmental Health Officers	*304*	*1358*	*18%*
Health Surveillance Assistants	*3,600*	*7,400*	*33%*

Staff per 100,000 population			
Malawi	*Tanzania*	*Botswana*	*S.Africa*
Physicians 1 .6*	*4.1*	*28.7*	*25.1*
Nurses 28.6	*85.2*	*241*	*140*

**8 if Clinical Officers are included*

As a stop gap measure a number of expatriate doctors have been recruited for district hospitals but this is not ideal. In any case, most patients continue to be seen and treated by Clinical Officers, Medical Assistants, Nurses, and attendants.

This is true in all medical fields. A survey showed that during 1993-95, in 18 District Hospitals, 75% of surgery was done by Clinical Officers and that 63% of all major operations were Caesarian Sections. This remains true and the appropriate and affordable Clinical Officer will remain the backbone of the health services for years to come.

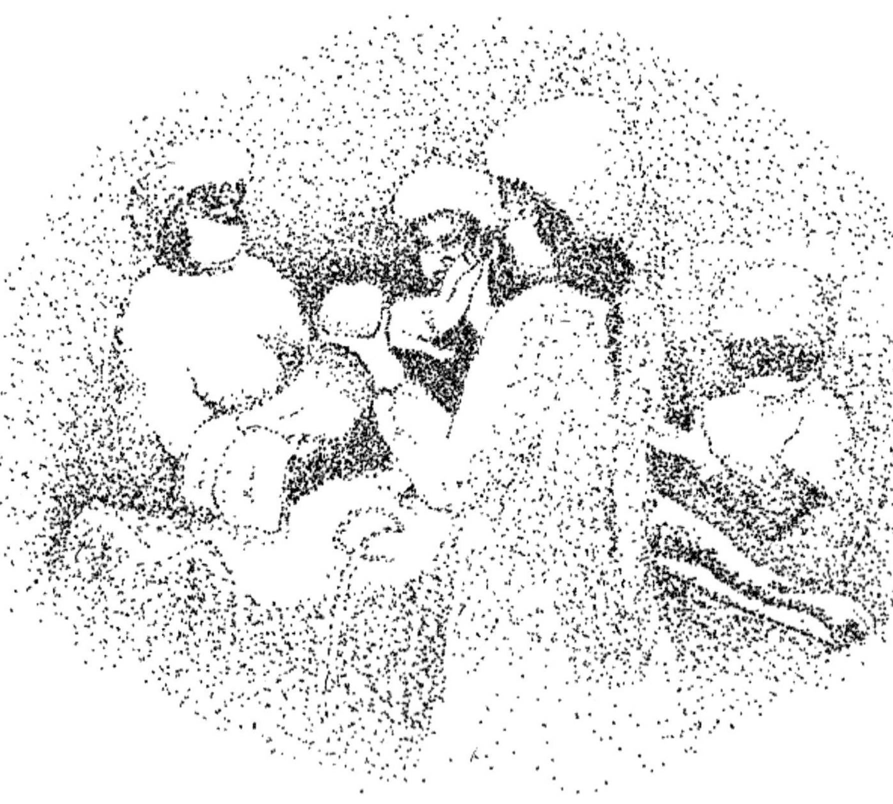

Caesarian Section, the commonest operation

Obstetric emergencies are displacing cold or elective surgery. Staff, theatre time, equipment and sutures have to be reserved, even though the elective surgery may be potentially life saving, such as repairing a hernia which could become obstructed. In a survey in one District Hospital in 1970 there were two Caesarian sections for every hernia repaired. By 2005 there were five.

Clinical Officers are trained in Blantyre, Lilongwe, and Malamulo (Adventist), now in increasing numbers. The century old dream of Dr. Laws for a Christian University at Livingstonia is being supported by donors. There will be appropriate training for health staff, teachers, and artisans. Mzuzu University is now starting new courses in Biomedical Sciences, Optometry, Dentistry, Pharmacy and Nursing. The problem will be retention of the graduates, as with doctors.

In the last 15 years several new hospitals have been built with donor funds. At Mzuzu in 2002, a 300 bedded Central Hospital was opened by the Taiwanese, who also continue to provide Specialists and other staff. In Blantyre, the Beit Trust/Cure hospital was set up in 2003, providing free orthopaedic care for children and paying facilities for adults.

Working there and at the College of Medicine, is Prof. N. Mkandawire, the first and only Malawian orthopaedic surgeon. In 2006 he was elected President of the College of Surgeons of East, Central, and Southern Africa. This body conducts exams so that postgraduate studies in surgery can now be carried out in Africa - not as before in the very different environment and pathologies of the US or UK.

Mission hospitals charge fees, have more clinical staff and fewer patients. Part of their staff salaries are paid by government. Many have funding from abroad (although this is decreasing) and have improved their buildings. They provide about 30% of health care in the country and 77% of the nurse training.

It is an anomaly that in areas served by these hospitals, patients have to pay for services and provide their own food. Fifteen years ago there were talks about introducing a cost recovery scheme for Government facilities - charging limited fees for services. This came to nothing because of political disquiet. But there are many points in its favour.

Most patients first go to herbalists or sing'angas, who charge. Treatment is more valued if paid for. If drugs are available free, they may be collected and then sold on by patients, and unnecessary visits to the overcrowded outpatient clinic are made. In neighbouring countries, 'free medical services' now mean that sick patients have to buy their own drugs, dressings and even intravenous fluids in the local market - a scenario that has been glimpsed in Malawi at times. Donors, politicians and patients object to paying medical fees - it seems unfair. But if administered with exemption for the very poor, it would undoubtedly improve hospital services.

"No one can shave your head in your absence" Malawian Minister implying that the Government is equally responsible for accepting policies from the Donors.

The Ministry of Health, with much donor assistance, is struggling to organize a more efficient way of funding and running health services. But donors do not always agree on policies in health, agriculture, and education etc. Aid to Malawi comes from many sources - from DFID in UK, UN Agencies, USAID, the EU, Germany, Taiwan, Japan and from smaller countries like Norway, Iceland and Ireland. 60% of government expenditure is from donor funds.

X-Ray equipment is being renewed and CT scanning is available in Blantyre for a fee. There are kidney dialysis machines in Lilongwe, but maintenance of hospital equipment is a problem. A unit has been formed for this but for spare parts and specialist repairs the country relies on South Africa.

All funds for health projects are put into one pot and the decentralized districts decide on its allocation. In the past year there has been a doubling or tripling of monthly health budgets to be spent in each district. The capacity for managing them is limited.

In a poor society, corruption is a temptation at all levels. Central Government has often not set a good example. Donors have helped set up an Anti-Corruption Bureau and insist on prosecution of culprits before more funds are released. Often 'tiddlers are caught and the sharks go free'. At a lower level poverty can lead to misuse and selling of drugs.

Disease

Spurred on by the AIDS epidemic, various research centres have been set up, by the UK Wellcome Trust and Liverpool School of Tropical Medicine, and several American Universities - John Hopkins, University of North Carolina, and others.

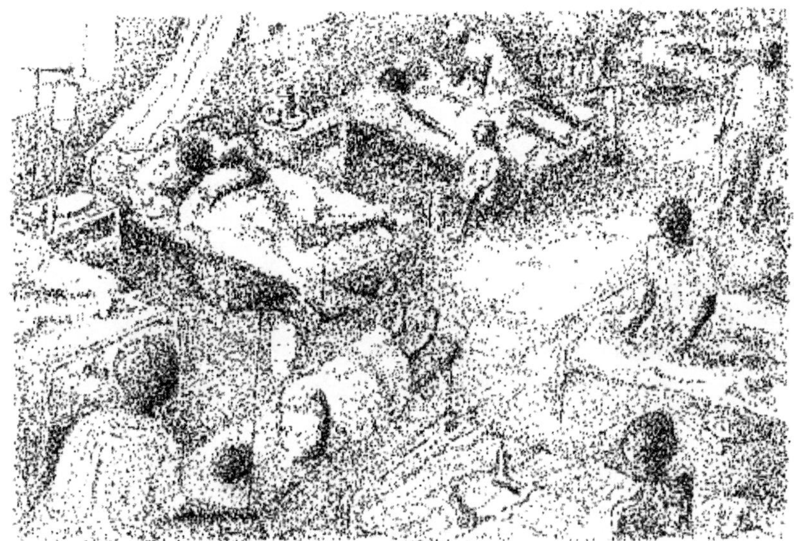

A new patient

Malaria is being studied and it continues to take a heavy toll about 5 million cases a year. In most district hospitals it is usual to see four or five infants having blood transfusions, which may save them from the severe anaemia caused by malaria. Subsidized mosquito nets have been widely distributed. Standard treatment using SP (Sulphadoxine pyrimethamine) has a 30% resistance rate. Quinine remains a standby but tragically is not always available. WHO hopes to introduce artemesin, (based on a plant) but there are fears resistance may develop to this expensive drug, which should be used in combination with other drugs.

Price of drugs limits their availability. Drug companies spend millions, and test hundreds, before a single effective drug is found and proved to be safe. They have to recoup their research and development costs. Patents protect them and prevent cheaper copies being made - until recently. New 'generic' drugs can now be made under licence in India, China and elsewhere for the poor world. Most of Malawi's drugs are sourced this way.

Some diseases only affect the poor so pharmaceutical companies see no profit in tackling them. **Sleeping Sickness** is one of these. The treatment remains toxic and based on arsenicals. In the 1990s there was a sudden increase in cases at Nkhota Kota hospital accounting for 11% of all hospital deaths at one time.

This followed a relaxation of the exclusion zone around the nearby game park, allowing farmers to encroach. In this century there has been an increase in cases at Rumphi hospital coming from the fringes of Vwaza Reserve. Some were villagers who had to use the nearby river because their borehole pump had failed (due to lack of simple maintenance - a constant story in Malawi). Others were fishermen, honey or wood gatherers, or poachers.

There is a dilemma. Tsetse flies protect wild animal game parks from encroachment by humans and cattle. Elephants, hippos, and other indigenous wild animals are protected species, but if they devastate crops, villagers take a different attitude. Man impacts on his environment everywhere and biodiversity suffers.

Even when cheap and effective drugs are available - as with praziquantel for **Bilharzia**, - may be often out of stock, largely due to incompetence, and occasionally dubious deals, somewhere along the line of supply.

Some diseases are declining. **Polio** seems to have been eliminated in Malawi and any suspicious cases of flaccid paralysis are tested. The world would have been free of this disease now were it not for the interruption of the vaccination programme in Nigeria due to unjustified fears over its effects. Malawi Against Polio, MAP, is now 'Malawi Against Physical Disabilities' and continues good work.

Leprosy is also declining due to the rifampicin drug programme and the armadillo vaccine trial by Lepra has been halted. The old Lepra centre at Chilumba on the northern lakeshore is now a Wellcome medical research unit. Research on TB and AIDS has been done with retrospective analysis of 40,000 blood samples collected in 1981-83 during a leprosy survey.

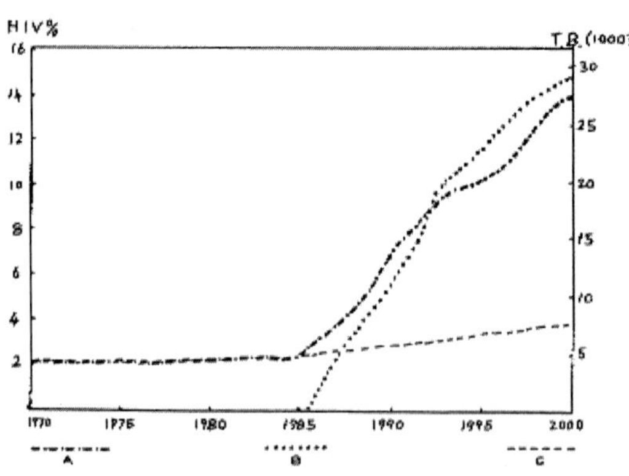

A) TB cases , B) HIV cases, C) Estimated TB cases without HIV

Tuberculosis is an increasing problem, 77% of cases are HIV-positive. The number of TB patients has increased threefold in twenty years. About a third of TB patients die within a few months of registration. Since 2001, DOTS (Directly Observed Treatment Short Course) has reduced in-patient stay. The family supervise the patient taking the drugs at home. The use of BCG (anti TB) vaccination has been widespread in the world for many years, but it has not proved very effective in Malawi. But Malawi continues to achieve a high level of childhood immunization against childhood diseases. The roll out of Anti-Retro Viral AIDS drugs benefits from the experience of the TB programme..

Laboratory services in Malawi are limited. District hospitals have technicians in their labs, which are now being upgraded by the UK. But only basic tests can be done. This includes collecting blood for transfusion, usually from family members or schools. There is always a shortage.

In 2004 the Malawi Blood Transfusion Service was set up with EU funds in Blantyre, to spread to other centres. The blood is screened and blood products are distributed. It does not reach all district hospitals. The programme is designed eventually to be handed over to the Ministry. If blood is easily available, the maternal and infant mortality can be halved.

Histopathology services are limited and not free. A diagnosis usually has to be made on clinical grounds only. **Kaposi's Sarcoma** remains the most common cancer, HIV related. It sometimes responds to chemotherapy, available officially only if the patient is HIV-positive. The childhood disease **Burkitt's Lymphoma** also responds well to chemotherapy and perhaps 50% of patients are cured. But the drugs are in short supply, sometimes funded only by individual donations

The incidence of **Breast Cancer** may be increasing but is nowhere near the very high incidence in the rich world. **Cervical cancer** remains common and usually presents at a late stage. There are a few efforts at cervical screening but the health services are too overburdened to take on this approach. Hope may come from a commercial vaccine against Human Papilloma Virus, known to be associated with the cancer. A trial of vaccinating pre-pubertal girls in the African situation is needed to prove its value here.

Maternal Mortality is now an alarming 1.2% and one in seven Malawian mothers can expect to die during a lifetime of childbearing.

Family planning has become more acceptable but supplies and staff are limited. Banja la Mtsogola supported by DFID and Marie Stopes International has opened thirty clinics, offering contraceptive and other health services for a small fee. With the motto "Children by Choice not Chance" Banja has outreach clinics for tubal ligation and consultations.

In 1992, the Association of Commonwealth Medical Associations meeting in Blantyre recommended that safe termination of pregnancy should be legalized in African countries. This would be especially valuable for HIV-positive women. Abortion is not yet legal in Malawi and unsafe abortions remain a common form of family planning with illness and death. 25% of gynaecological beds are occupied by girls with incomplete abortions (not necessarily induced). One survey showed that half of their pregnancies were not wanted.

When supplementary food was given to pregnant mothers in Chikwawa district in 1996, the already poor local contraceptive uptake decreased significantly. Women became pregnant to qualify for free food. The World Food Programme has withdrawn from some areas. The long term effects of overpopulation were being compounded and communities made unsustainable.

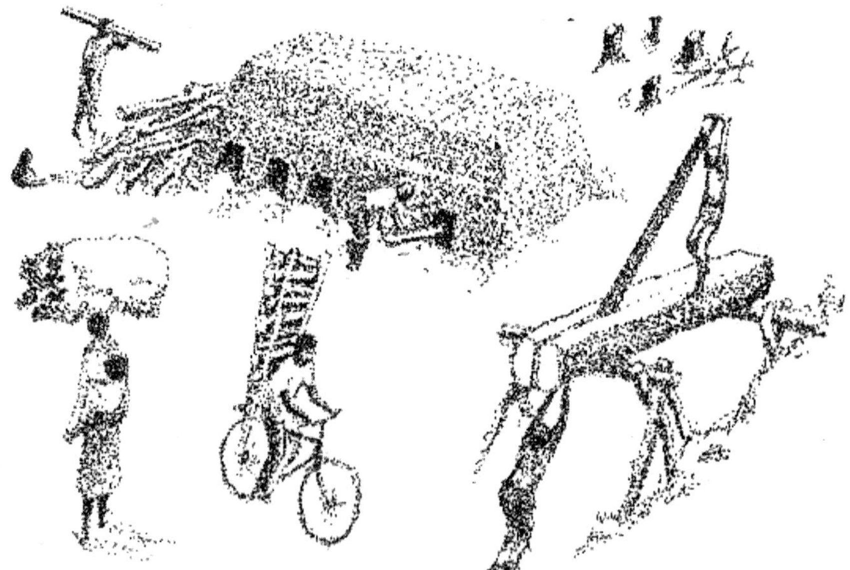

Trees must be felled. Brick Kiln   Pit Sawing   Logs and Charcoal for Fuel

Population and Environment

Malawi is remains a beautiful country, but trees are being felled at an unsustainable rate. Previously forested hills are now bare. Trees must be cut for fuel and cooking, burning bricks, and to sell as charcoal. There is no alternative for most Malawians. More land is cleared for cultivation. As a result, fertile top soil runs off in the rainy season into the streams and rivers and then into Lake Malawi, where silt damages fish breeding grounds. The hydroelectric stations on the Shire River which provide electric power for the country are threatened by siltation and poor maintenance.

Human encroachment on animal spaces worldwide has resulted in cross-species transfer of viruses, notably HIV from primates, also Bird Flu, SARS, Lassa Fever, Ebola, and Rift Valley fever. Perhaps this is an attempt by nature to restore its balance, upset by three centuries of habitat and biodiversity destruction caused by human expansion?

We have not been able to limit our numbers by rational decisions, so fate imposes. Conflicts over land, food, water, soil and air pollution inevitably occur. Increasing unemployment, drug and alcohol abuse can result in early deaths and suicides.

Before 1992, by Presidential decree, the term 'family planning' could not be used. Overpopulation was denied, birth control had to be called 'child spacing'. In 1992 the Malawi Medical Association discussed population issues. Alarming predictions were made, but the urgency for action has been overtaken by a resigned fatalism. A few people still campaign within Malawi for limitations in family size. In 2006 the fertility rate is 6 children born per woman, and annual population growth rate is 2.4%.

Rich countries, with low fertility, do not have this problem. But their profligate use of global resources damages the planet - especially with fossil fuels emitting carbon dioxide. This causes the greenhouse effect in the upper atmosphere and global warming. A Malawian produces 1/150th of the 'carbon footprint' of a Briton. Yet the agriculture and lives of poor Africans will be far more affected by climate change. As a result of this Malawi has recently experienced more floods and droughts.

It is not enough for the guilty rich to give aid to the poor. Let us hope they will lead the way and help to develop clean energy, including nuclear power, before it is too late.

The health of us all now depends on the temperature of the globe

<u>In Memoriam   Malawi's Forest Trees and Environment</u>

Headline from a full page newspaper advertisement in 2005, an appeal signed by twelve important local organizations with a request to the Government to: **introduce and enforce a strong family planning policy which would reduce the high population growth rate with the long term objective of of having a population that is in balance with the available natural resources.**

Some selected references for further reading

Broadhead R.L., Mvula A.S. "Creating a Medical School for Malawi" BMJ August 17th 2002

Crampin A. et al "Long term follow up of HIV-positive and HIV-negative individuals in rural Malawi" AIDS 2002; 16, 1545-1550

Dallabetta G. et al "High Social Economic as a Risk Factor for HIV-1 Control" Journal of Infectious Diseases 1993; 167,36-42

Fenton P. "District Surgery in Malawi" East and Central African Journal of Surgery; June 1997

Harries A.D., Saliponi F.M. et al "High death rates among health care workers and teachers in Malawi" Trans. Roy. Soc. Trop. Med. Hyg. 1996;

King Maurice "Primary Mother Care and Population" Spiegle Press 2003

King Michael and Elspeth "The Great Rift - Africa, Surgery, AIDS, Aid" ISBN   0-9539290-0-0

Lavy C.B.D. "Global Need in Orthopaedics" Brit. Orth. Assoc. Glasgow September 2006

Lewis D.K. et al "Prevalence and indicators of HIV and AIDS among adults admitted to medical and surgical wards in Blantyre, Malawi" Malawi Medical Journal 2001

McCormack Grace et al "Early Evolution of the Human Immune- Deficiency Virus Subtype C Epidemic in rural Malawi" Journal of Virology Dec. 2002, 12890-12899

Molyneux M.and E. - Malawi Research Abstracts in Malawi Medical Journal, January 2005

Ratsma Y.E.C. Malawi Medical Journal 1993 - devoted to Family Planning and Population problems

Sangala V. "Safe Abortion - A Woman's Right" Tropical Doctor July 2005

Taha T. et al "Mortality after first year of life among human immuno-deficiency virus infected and uninfected children" Pediatr. Infect. Dis. 1999